THE CANCER NUTRITION CENTER HANDBOOK

An Essential Guide for Cancer Patients
And their Families

BY

CAROLYN KATZIN, MS, CNS, MNT
CERTIFIED NUTRITION SPECIALIST

This publication contains the opinions and ideas of the author. It is intended to provide helpful and informative material on the subjects addressed in this publication. It is sold with the understanding that the author and publisher are not engaged in rendering medical, health, psychological, or any other kind of personal professional services in the book. The nutrition advice is intended to support not to take the place of any medical treatment.

The author and publisher specifically disclaim all responsibility for any liability, loss, or risk, personal or otherwise, that is incurred as a consequence, directly or indirectly, of the use and application of any of the contents of this book.

Copyright ©2001, 2003, 2006, 2011 by Carolyn Katzin

ISBN 10 0-9651736-3-1
ISBN 13 978-0-9651736-3-6

This book or parts thereof, may not be reproduced in any form without permission from the publisher, exceptions are made for brief excerpts used for published reviews.

Printed in the United States of America
      10 9 8 7 6 5 4 3 2 1

Library of Congress Cataloging-in-Publication Data
      Is available from the Publisher

For my mother and father

Acknowledgements

With many thanks to all who made this book possible.
Thank you to my daughter, Zara Fletcher for her excellent editing.
Thank you to Betsy Carver for her expert assistance in layout.

CONTENTS

Introduction and how to use this book	1
Nutrition guidelines for everyone	2
Eating to reduce your risk of cancer	3
Standard Serving Size / Healthy Body Weight	5
Three stages in a cycle of nutrition and cancer	6
Personalized nutrition	7

Nutrition during treatment
    Preparing for treatment
    During treatment
    After treatment - survivorship
	8

Oral health during treatment	9
Skin health during treatment	11
Some drug specific nutrition advice	12
Radiation treatment and nutrition	19
Some supplements and helpful foods	19
Some important reminders	20
Herbs and surgery warnings	21
Foods for health	21

Suggestions for handling treatment side effects
    For chewing and swallowing difficulties
    For dealing with diarrhea
    For dealing with constipation
    For dealing with nausea and/or vomiting
    For dealing with loss of appetite
	22

Eating to provide maximum immunity	24

Sugar	25
Inflammatory processes and cancer	26
Digestive enzymes	27
If someone you love has cancer	27
Sample food choices	28
Some diet suggestions	29
To increase calories	
To increase protein	
To increase cancer fighting phytonutrients	
To increase iron	
To increase magnesium	
To increase zinc	
For general blood building properties	
My Daily Food Guide	31
Helpful recipes	32
If your mouth is sore	
If you are constipated	
If you have diarrhea	
If your white cell count is low	
Recipes	
Appetizers	33
Soups	39
Beans, Pasta and Rice	52
Fish	72
Poultry	86
Vegetables and Vegetarian Dishes	91
Desserts and Comfort Foods	109
Beverages and Smoothies	124
Recipe index	144
Handbook text index	146
Bibliography and further reading	151

INTRODUCTION

In 1986, I began working with participants (people who had been diagnosed with cancer but were not defined by that diagnosis) at The Wellness Community in Santa Monica. Each Friday, I would prepare lunch and share why food was especially important. I explained how eating well would improve their resilience and help them to face the challenges that lay ahead. The late Harold Benjamin who founded The Wellness Community after his wife was diagnosed with breast cancer introduced the "patient active" concept and was a wonderful mentor and inspiration to me and thousands of others. At that time I was asked to volunteer for the American Cancer Society and so began an amazing journey of learning and teaching. Over the past twenty-three years, my nutrition practice has specialized in assisting those faced with cancer. I have learned that good nutrition is empowering and even healing.

I developed a nutrition guide for participants of The Wellness Community and have published three earlier editions which have been for sale on my website www.cancernutrition.com since its launch in 1997. This guide is a living document and I owe much to the input I have received from so many cancer patients and their loved ones. I thank you all from the bottom of my heart.

The information in this handbook is arranged to assist those newly diagnosed, those undergoing treatment and for survivors and all who wish for health. The Cycle of Nutrition and Cancer describes how during active treatment it is often difficult to eat an ideal diet due to poor appetite, fatigue and also because this type of eating plan is usually high in dietary fiber and may take a lot of effort to chew. Harsh textured food is damaging to delicate digestive tissues for example, especially those in the mouth. During this time soft textured food is most helpful. In my opinion, the most important thing to do is to maintain a healthy weight and stay strong. This may mean eating foods that are higher in healthy oils or fats like avocado and olives and selecting foods that are easy to digest. I call this the Expedient Diet. However, as the acute treatment time is usually short and cyclical this is a time to choose tasty foods you like and want to eat above all. Later on, you can make up for any possible nutritional imbalances by eating especially beneficial foods and supplements in, what I term, the Regenerative phase of the cycle. Many people have thanked me for providing this charted course of nutrition as it has helped them to fend off well-meaning but often bossy or intrusive dietary suggestions from friends and family. You can simply tell them about the Cycle of Nutrition for Cancer Patients and that you are in your Expedient Diet phase when you reach for the only thing you fancy, even if it may not be a healthy item in isolation.

My desire is that this book and the recipes at the end will assist you and your family in making this journey a little easier.

Carolyn Katzin
Los Angeles, June, 2011

NUTRITION GUIDELINES for everyone

The National Cancer Institute and the American Cancer Society estimate that 35% of all cancers are linked to diet. Physical activity is also vitally important and when combined with a healthy diet, they both provide the best opportunity for staying healthy. Fresh, wholesome food is crucial for a healthy immune system.

1. Choose at least five servings (or about 1½ pounds) of vegetables and fruit each day. Many studies show a decreased risk of lung, prostate, bladder, esophageal and stomach cancers with plenty of fruits and vegetables in the diet. Dark green, yellow and orange types of vegetables are the richest in protective botanical factors also called phytonutrients. Black raspberries (see cover) are especially rich in these as are blueberries and dark red grapes are also rich in antioxidants, anticarcinogens and anti-inflammatory botanical factors. I call these the three A's. Choose most of the foods you eat from plant sources. Choose whole grains as opposed to refined or processed ones as they have more B vitamins, zinc, magnesium and other important nutrients. Choose beans often as an alternative to meat. Select organically grown produce whenever you can.

2. Limit your intake of high fat foods, particularly from animal sources. High fat diets have been associated with an increase in the risk of cancers of the colon and rectum, prostate and endometrium. The association with breast cancer is weaker. Choose foods low in animal fat by replacing fat-rich foods with fruits, vegetables, grains and beans. Eat smaller portions and select non-fat or low-fat (1%) dairy products. Select lean cuts of meat and bake or broil using marinades which reduce nitrosamine formation rather than frying. Choose fish, seafood and poultry often. Healthy oils do not need to be restricted; these include oily fish, olives, avocado, nuts and seeds. These are beneficial.

3. Be physically active: achieve and maintain a healthy weight. Physical activity can help to protect against some cancers and assist in recovery. At least thirty minutes of moderate activity on most days of the week is recommended for well being. Physical activity stimulates bowel health and may play a part in normalizing hormone levels and reducing prostate and breast cancer risks. Recent studies have suggested a protection from skin cancer which may also be related to vitamin D due to the action of sunlight on the skin.

4. Limit consumption of alcoholic beverages, if you drink at all. In countries where alcohol consumption is high (more than two drinks a day) oral and esophageal cancers are more common. There is a more than additive effect with smoking. Moderate intakes of wine or beer with food are associated with improved cardiovascular health and add to the enjoyment of a meal. The American Cancer Society recommends no alcohol at all if you have a family history of breast cancer.

Remember that **moderation and variety** are the keys to a healthy diet and lifestyle.

EATING TO REDUCE YOUR RISK OF CANCER

- Eat fresh fruit and a salad every day. Use olive oil and lemon juice or balsamic vinegar as a salad dressing. Sprinkle a few pine nuts (pignolas), walnuts or almonds on top of your salad for healthy omega-3 fatty acids, B vitamins and dietary fiber. Hard boiled egg white increases the protein.

- Eat at least 5 servings of fruits and vegetables each day. For most people this means simply adding one more serving. 8-10 servings are even better for you as they are rich in the three A's Antioxidants, Anti-inflammatories and Anticarcinogens.

- Half a cup of berries (fresh or frozen) has as much cancer-fighting antioxidant activity as 5 servings of most other fruits and vegetables.

- Eat high fiber, folate rich beans and peas 3 or more times a week. Vary your types of beans: black, mung, adzuki, garbanzo, kidney, soy, green beans and peas.

- Wash fruits and vegetables well and eat with the skin on whenever possible.
  The skin and just under the skin are where most of the nutrients and fiber are.

- Cabbage (all types), broccoli, Brussels sprouts, bok choy and other cruciferous vegetables are particularly rich in cancer fighting phytonutrients or botanical factors.

- Try tofu, soy milk and cheese, edamame and other soy foods for a variety of cancer fighting factors. Limit soy phytoestrogens to no more than 30 mg per day if you have estrogen receptor positive breast cancer. Soy sauce, veggie burgers are fine. Soy sauce, miso and soy oil have very little or no phytoestrogens.

- Add half a cup of wheat germ to your breakfast cereals for added B vitamins, vitamin E and dietary fiber.

- Use instant oatmeal in meat loaf recipes for added fiber.

- Include fresh fruit or whole juices often. If drinking juices make sure they are 100% juice as some labels can be misleading.

- Include spinach often. It is rich in cancer fighting nutrients. Wash well and eat small, fresh leaves if possible or lightly steamed.

- Include watercress often. It is rich in beta carotene and other phytonutrients.

- Use garlic when cooking. Garlic was mentioned by Hippocrates 2500 years ago as a cancer fighting food.

- When using lemons and limes, remember to twist the zest for the essential oils in the rind. These are particularly good cancer fighters.

- Eat cantaloupe, pomegranates, blueberries, apricots, spinach and carrots often for beta carotene and other cancer fighting phytonutrients.

- Eat watermelon, pink grapefruit, tomato paste in your sauce and fresh tomatoes often for lycopene and other cancer fighting phytonutrients.

- Eat green, red and yellow bell peppers often for Vitamin C and other cancer fighting nutrients. Slice and add to salads or chop finely into other dishes.

- Always include lettuce and tomato in your sandwiches. If possible, ask for peppers and onions too.

- Eat fish often. Choose wild salmon often. Tuna, halibut, herrings and sardines are all good choices. Remember to vary your types of fresh fish. Many people who eat fish regularly have a reduced risk of heart disease, stroke and possibly some forms of cancer too.

- Eat red grapes and drink red grape juice or small quantities of red wine (unless you have breast cancer in the family when the American Cancer Society suggests you do not drink alcohol at all). Red grapes contain a cancer fighting nutrient resveratrol as well as other healthful phytonutrients.

STANDARD SERVING SIZES

Fruits
    1 medium apple, banana, orange
    Half a cup of chopped, cooked or canned fruit
    3/4 cup of 100% fruit juice

Vegetables
    1 cup of raw vegetables
    Half a cup of cooked vegetables
    Half a cup of chopped raw vegetables
    3/4 cup vegetable juice

Grains
    1 slice bread
    1 ounce ready-to-eat cereal
    Half a cup of cooked cereal, rice, or pasta

Beans and nuts
    Half a cup cooked beans
    2 tablespoons peanut or almond butter
    1/3 cup nuts

Dairy foods and eggs
    1 cup milk or yogurt
    One and a half ounces of natural cheese

Meat and fish
    2-3 ounces lean meat, poultry or fish

HEALTHY BODY WEIGHT

Increasing evidence suggests that a healthy body weight is very important to your quality of life. Body Mass Index (BMI) is the ratio of your height to your weight, and ideally, should be between 19 and 24.9. A BMI above 25 is considered overweight and above 30 is considered obese. A pear rather than an apple shape is also linked to health but this tends to be genetic and difficult to alter. A healthy waist size is considered to be 40 inches or under for men (usually related to a pant size two inches smaller) and 35 inches or under for women. Divide your height by two and this should be your upper waist size. Central adiposity or belly fat is associated with higher risks of inflammation and this may be particularly important if you have been diagnosed with cancer. Belly fat is responsive to exercise especially core type such as yoga or Pilates. Deep breathing type of energy work is helpful especially when you feel fatigued.

THREE STAGES IN A CYCLE OF NUTRITION AND CANCER

1. **Preventive Nutrition (when you feel well)**
   - Fats or oils from fish, nuts and seeds need not be restricted. Saturated fats from meats, dairy products or hydrogenated oils should be restricted to less than 10% of total energy intake.
   - Rich in foods from plant sources such as whole grains, beans, starchy root vegetables, nuts, green, leafy vegetables and darkly pigmented fruits.
   - Reasonable in protein; two servings daily (about the size of a deck of cards) of fish, lean meat, poultry or one cup of mixed beans and rice.
   - Plenty of antioxidants and phytonutrients or botanical factors found in whole grains, beans, vegetables and many fruits. Dark colored items are richest sources. Eat some frequently.
   - Moderate quantities overall. Stay active to maintain a steady weight.
   - Wide variety of foods, especially seasonal fruits and vegetables. Eat a minimum of 5 servings each day, 8-10 servings are recommended.

2. **During Treatment (Expedient Diet)**
   - Frequent, easily-digested, small meals of sufficient energy to maintain body weight.
   - Stay as active as possible. Try walking, stretching, yoga and stress reducing types of activities.
   - One more serving per day of protein; use protein powder for smoothies or include hard boiled eggs on salads or add egg whites, more fish and poultry at meal times.
   - Few dairy products due to possible lactose-intolerance which may develop; symptoms include abdominal discomfort and diarrhea. Live culture yogurt or hard cheese are usually okay.
   - Avoid gas-producing foods such as insufficiently cooked beans or excessive amounts of the cabbage family. Use digestive enzymes to reduce gas and bloating.
   - Avoid highly spiced foods, unless they agree with you.
   - Be especially vigilant with food safety.
   - Avoid high dose antioxidant supplements.

3. **Regenerative Nutrition (as you recover and transition back to Preventive [Survivorship] Nutrition)**
   - As with Preventive Nutrition but with a special focus on the nutrients needed for regenerating the immune system, for instance Vitamins B, C, E, selenium and zinc.
   - Be physically active, introducing more varieties and intensity of exercise as you feel better. Use breathing exercises to help balance your acid/base balance and receive full benefits of being active even when you are fatigued.
   - At least 10 servings of fruits and vegetables each day. Try 100% fruit or vegetable juices but remember to wash all produce well. Food safety is still a vitally important aspect of your recovery.
   - Reintroduce milk and lactose containing dairy products slowly.
   - Include a daily antioxidant rich multivitamin and mineral supplement.

PERSONALIZED NUTRITION

In 2001 the first draft of the human genome was completed and now personalized nutrition is fast becoming a reality. By the time you read this you may already have had your DNA analyzed to learn how fast you metabolize certain medications. If you are taking more than three medications on a regular basis I encourage you to learn more about your liver enzyme profiles. Targeted cancer therapies now rely on genetic testing of tumor tissue to learn which would be most effective. Learning about our genome is rather like Google Earth focusing in to key features and landmarks. This is a new era of medicine and health and the benefits are only just being felt.

In addition to how efficiently your body metabolizes medications and herbs you may also wish to learn more about how you handle the approximately 23,000 different food components you may be exposed to on any typical day. Common variations in our molecular identity or genetic code occur very frequently and offer insights into how well you may handle certain foods. For instance, you may have variations that affect your insulin sensitivity. Once you know this you can choose low glycemic foods (those that release sugar slowly into your blood stream), eat small, frequent meals and choose healthy oils which also slow down stomach emptying. For more details on personalized nutrition please visit my site www.thednadiet.com

For most people the Mediterranean Diet is recommended as being the healthiest; it is rich in colorful vegetables and fruits especially tomatoes and citrus fruits. Fish is eaten frequently (at least twice a week) and red meat is limited. Olives, almonds, walnuts, pistachios and other sources of healthy oils are eaten frequently and salads are dressed with extra virgin olive oil. Beans (fava, garbanzo, green beans, etc.) are also eaten frequently providing B vitamins and dietary fiber. Most of the recipes in this book are based on the Mediterranean Diet and provide colorful botanical benefits.

Red grapes and red wine are rich in resveratrol which is a powerful antioxidant. Many people enjoy a glass of red wine or red grape juice with their meal. I suggest selecting organic wines whenever possible. Dark chocolate is another excellent source of resveratrol and other antioxidants. Again, organic is best. Try a small square as an afternoon pick me up.

NUTRITION DURING TREATMENT

If you have been diagnosed with cancer, eating well is one of the most important things for you to consider as part of your whole treatment regimen. A simple rule of thumb is to maintain a steady body weight throughout treatment. This means neither gaining too much, nor losing too much weight (fluctuations of more than 5lbs per week for an average sized adult). If you are overweight at the beginning of treatment it is safe to lose about a pound a week but this probably isn't the time to embark on a weight loss diet. Nurture yourself with a wide range of healthful things not just food as you build up your resilience and navigate your own personal journey. Many people find this a great time to participate in creative projects for example.

Preparing for Treatment:

Surgery: Eat a low fat (less than 25% of total calories), high protein diet of two or three protein rich foods such as fish, eggs, chicken or lean meat; beans and rice if vegetarian. Supplement with a multivitamin and mineral supplement containing DAILY VALUE amounts. An additional supplement containing 500 mg vitamin C with bioflavonoids taken every 8 hours for 2 days before surgery and for a week afterwards may be beneficial to healing. Stop all supplements of vitamins E and K, evening primrose, borage or fish oils one week before surgery as these may cause thinning of the blood. Do not take any herbs without informing your medical team as they may interfere with other medications. Avoid grapefruit juice as this may affect liver enzyme clearance of some medications.
Radiation: Usual preventive nutrition diet but no supplements beyond usual RDA level multivitamin of vitamin C or E.
Chemo: Eat a low fat, high carbohydrate diet the day before chemotherapy. No supplements on day of treatment.

During Treatment:

Surgery: According to your medical professionals' protocols.
Radiation: Extra carbohydrate calories: try green tea or Siberian ginseng for energy.
Chemo: Avoid eating your favorite foods within 24 hours of treatment to avoid negative associations with them at a later time. Eat a low fat (less than 3 tablespoons or 40 grams total fat or oil per day), high complex carbohydrate diet. Most of your energy should come from whole grain breads, cereals, beans, fruits and vegetables with an additional serving of protein. White meat chicken, fish and eggs are easy to digest. Protein powder based smoothies are also good. Avoid more than 100% Daily Value of antioxidant supplements as these may interfere with clearance of the chemotherapy medications.

After Treatment:

Surgery: High protein diet; three servings daily of lean meat, poultry, fish or eggs or add in a protein smoothie. Regular supplements as above. Include an antioxidant supplement.
Radiation: High protein and energy diet. Lactose-free and relatively low in simple sugars (sucrose or honey) to avoid intestinal discomfort or bloating.
Chemo: See next section for details of specific drug/nutrient interactions.

NUTRITION AND CHEMOTHERAPY

General Nutritional Advice

Chemotherapy today has fewer side effects than in the past. However in order to achieve its goal of killing cancer cells there are still challenges to overcome. A good way to minimize these side effects is to select a high protein, low sugar diet that is rich in anti inflammatory nutrients such as omega-3 fatty acids (from microalgae DHA fortified foods for example) and natural salicylates such as found in culinary herbs and spices including oregano and turmeric.

ORAL HEALTH DURING TREATMENT

The mouth is home to some of the fastest dividing cells in the body. There are also an estimated 6 billion bacteria and other microbes from at least 600 different species that live in this environment. Since the introduction of 16S RNA probes there has been a much better understanding of how the microbiota or microbial flora in the mouth behave both in normal conditions and when disturbed such as by radiation directly to the area. Scientists in Switzerland have recently discovered that bacteria in the human mouth play a role in producing the flavors of some foods with saliva trapping aromas to modulate longer lasting flavors. From a nutritional perspective there are some other important factors to consider:

1) Lysine to arginine ratio - 500 mg L-lysine is helpful in reducing risk of cold sores. Elderberries are also antiviral as are alpha and beta glucans (in medicinal mushrooms for example)

2) L-glutamine may also be helpful as a topical liquid (10 grams glutamine powder dissolved in warm water and swished then swallowed three times daily). Some people also suggest 15 grams orally for lower digestive health during treatment up to twice daily

3) Avoid sticky, sugary foods such as caramels or jelly beans as these encourage yeast over-growth (oral thrush)

4) Avoid high acid foods and beverages such as orange juice as this can burn especially if the mouth is already sore

5) Balancing oral pH with alkaline rinses (non alcoholic type)

6) Rinse frequently with warm saline solution

7) Maintain a high salivary flow with sugarless gum/candy

8) Ensure a regular intake of soft foods including high nutrient density protein drinks, e.g. MRM Natural Gainer (whey) protein powder with probiotics and digestive enzymes

9) Ensure nutrient intake is continued throughout the 24 hour period with late night beverages such as papaya or guava nectar during the night followed by rinsing with saline

10) Alcohol and tobacco use should be avoided completely

Foods to Select

- Select soft, bland, non-acidic types of foods
- Ice cream (try Häagen Dazs® 5 a new version with high quality ingredients including ginger flavor). Allow to warm a little at room temperature or on defrost setting in microwave for softer texture
- Soft fruits including apple sauce or apricot, guava or pear nectars
- Mashed potatoes or sweet potatoes
- Cream of wheat, rice or other cooked smooth texture cereals
- Eggs, soft boiled, scrambled, omelets, etc.
- Yogurt (Greek style, full fat for example)
- Cottage cheese and sour cream
- Custards, puddings and mousses (made with gelatin)
- Nut butters
- Avocado
- Smooth texture foods – baby food portion size and texture is good

Foods to Avoid

- Avoid any rough, dry or harsh textured foods such as popcorn, pretzels, nuts
- Acidic foods such as lemon, orange or grapefruit or their juices
- Hard texture foods such as raw carrots, celery or hard apple
- Pickles
- Salad dressings with vinegar (unless cream type)
- Toffees or caramels

Suggestions

- Use a numbing type of mouthwash (non alcoholic)
- Rinse often with lightly salted water
- Maintain good dental hygiene using soft rotating brush, e.g. Rotadent®
- Use aloe vera juice or concentrate if very sore; aloe gel is a good addition to mouthwash
- Swill with antacid, e.g. Maalox
- Avoid very hot or very cold foods

Check to be sure that you don't needlessly struggle with constipation for example by selecting high fiber foods and including prune juice or other natural gentle laxatives. Several newer agents have constipation as a side effect.

Hydration is crucially important. Make sure you drink plenty of fluids in water, soups and unsweetened juices. Keep rehydration fluids on hand. A simple home-made remedy is to add a pinch of salt and a teaspoon of sugar to a cup of water. During chemotherapy it is easy to become dehydrated rapidly; fatigue is usually the first sign. Always contact your oncology health care team immediately if you suspect this.

Please ask your physician or oncologist to check your Vitamin D blood levels. This is becoming a very important nutrient (also a hormone) and some people have a very high requirement because of their genetic profile. This requires medical supervision to achieve optimal levels. If you are taking adjuvant therapies that affect your bone density such as aromatase inhibitors or other estrogen modulators then this is particularly important. Without ideal Vitamin D levels you won't be able to absorb or use calcium supplements effectively.

Below is an example of how to reduce or minimize possible side effects associated with EGFR inhibitors. As more chemotherapy agents become available that are individually tailored for specific cancers there will be more personalizing of your program using the new concept of 4P health – Personalized, Predictive, Preventative and Participatory (LeRoy Hood). Please contact me for a personalized nutrition consultation to expand upon your genetic test results. Carolyn@carolynkatzin.com

SKIN HEALTH DURING TREATMENT

Many newer chemotherapy agents including EGFR inhibitors such as Cetuximab (Erbitux) may trigger a skin rash in certain people. This is most likely due to a delayed T-cell response and is thought to indicate effectiveness of the reaction. Foods that may exacerbate this include psoralens which react with ultraviolet light or radiation treatment and cause a rash which becomes pigmented in its later stages. This mechanism is sometimes used to treat the unpigmented patches of skin in patients with vitiligo.

In order to minimize your risk of a rash avoid juicing large quantities of foods from the Apiacea (Umbelliferae) plant family:
- Celery, *Apium graveolens*
- Parsnip, *Pastinaca sativa*
- Parsley
- Fennel
- Anise
- Caraway
- Chervil
- Cumin
- Coriander/cilantro
- Carrot
- *Angelica archangelica* or *A.sinensis* (also known as Dong Quai in Chinese medicine)

Lime juice may also provoke a skin rash reaction in some people. Citrus fruit stimulates liver enzyme activity. Other chemotherapies that are associated with rash after sun exposure include 5-FU (fluorouracil), Methotrexate and Dacarbazine (DTIC or DTIC-Dome). If you don't have any rash symptoms then you probably won't have any problems eating these foods but if you do have a rash, it makes sense to avoid them and see if the rash improves.

Drink plenty of fluids - at least two liters total, with most of it coming from clear liquids such as water, apple juice, clear broths or Jell-o®. Avoid caffeine containing liquids such as tea, coffee and colas as these are dehydrating. Eat small quantities of food rather than large meals for easier digestion. Eat crackers, Melba toast, pasta and baked potatoes if you feel nauseated. Use the concept of the Expedient Diet and make up for eating less healthily, if needed, when you have more strength.

Eat avocado often as it is an excellent source of calories, essential fatty acids, potassium and glutathione, unless contraindicated (if on Procarbazine or other medication requiring a low tyramine diet).

SOME DRUG SPECIFIC NUTRITIONAL ADVICE

Abraxane, paclitaxel, taxol	Avoid caffeine, avoid grapefruit juice. DHA may be helpful. Bland foods. Drink extra fluids. Extra protein (include a smoothie for example)
Accutane, isotretinoin	Avoid alcohol; avoid sugar; eat low saturated animal fat diet; drink plenty of fluids. Do not take additional vitamin A as this increases toxicity potential
Adriamycin, doxorubicin,	Drink extra fluids; eat foods rich in B vitamins particularly riboflavin (see above)
Adrucil, fluorouracil, 5-FU	Drink extra fluids; eat foods rich in B vitamins
Afinitor, everolimus	Soft diet. Avoid acidic, spicy or salty foods
Alkeran, melphalan, L-PAM	Drink extra fluids
Alimta, pemetrexed	Vitamin B-12 and folate usually given at the same time. Avoid caffeine and alcohol. Avoid foods high in salicylates (see list below)
Arimidex, anastrozole	Calcium, magnesium and vitamin D
Aromasin, exemestane	Avoid high fat foods; exercise regularly to minimize possible weight gain side effect; eat foods rich in calcium and magnesium (dairy foods, broccoli, nuts and seeds). Avoid soy foods rich in phytoestrogens such as edamame, soy nuts and soy milk
Arranon, nelarabine	Drink extra fluids. Eat bland, soluble fiber rich diet to maintain regular bowel activity (prevent diarrhea or constipation)
Arzerra, ofatumumab	Include more protein
Avastin, bevacizumab	High fiber foods may be helpful to avoid constipation which so sometimes occurs. Apple sauce and oatmeal if diarrhea occurs

Bexxar, tositumomab	Extra protein, e.g. whey smoothie
Blenoxane, bleomycin,	Bland foods
Busulfex, busulfan, Myleran	Drink extra fluids; eat foods rich in B vitamins
Campath, alemtuzumab	Drink extra fluids. Eat soft, bland foods
Camptosar, irinotecan	Avoid grapefruit juice. Avoid lactose and high sugar foods; avoid laxatives (wheat bran, rhubarb, figs, etc.) Choose apple sauce.
Carmustine, BCNU, BiCNU	Bland foods; avocado
Carboplatin and cisplatin	Avoid purine rich foods (liver, caviar, sardines, anchovies) Eat plenty of magnesium, potassium and zinc rich foods (whole grains, nuts). Drink extra fluids. Avoid grapefruit juice which may lower the drug effectiveness. Avoid fish oil supplements
Casodex, bicalutamide	Avoid body building supplements that may contain plant forms of testosterone such as Tribulus terrestris as these reduce effectiveness of the medication
CeeNU, lomustine,	Bland foods; avocado
Cerubine, daunorubicin	Drink extra fluids; eat foods rich in B vitamins, particularly riboflavin (milk, lean meat, egg yolks, wheat germ)
Cytarabine, cytosine arabinoside	Drink extra fluids. Eat soft, bland foods. Fatty foods may increase nausea
Cytoxan, cyclophosphamide	Drink extra fluids. Avoid alcohol; eat bland and low fat foods. Avoid turmeric and curcumin as it may interfere with drug effectiveness
DepoCyt, liposomal Ara-C	Drink extra fluids. Eat soft, bland foods. Fatty foods may increase nausea
DITC-Dome, dacarbazine	Drink extra fluids; bland foods; avocado
Doxil, doxorubicin liposomal	Drink extra fluids (urine may turn pink)
Efudex, fluorouracil, 5-FU	Drink extra fluids; eat foods rich in B vitamins
Ellence, epirubicin chloride	Drink extra fluids (urine may turn pink)
Eloxatin, oxaliplatin	Drink extra fluids. Avoid cold foods or ice
Elspar, asparaginase, BAN	Drink extra fluids; consume extra calories
Erbitux, cetuximab	Eat magnesium, calcium and potassium rich foods. Avoid caffeine. Eat small, easy to digest meals (avoid fatty, spicy or acidic foods)

Eulexin, flutamide	Avoid body building supplements that may contain plant forms of testosterone such as Tribulus terrestris as these reduce effectiveness of the medication
Evista, raloxifene	Avoid high fat foods; exercise regularly to minimize possible weight gain side effect; eat foods rich in calcium and magnesium (dairy foods, broccoli, nuts and seeds). Avoid soy foods rich in phytoestrogens such as edamame, soy nuts and soy milk
Fareston, toremifene	Avoid soy foods rich in phytoestrogens such as edamame, soy nuts and soy milk
Faslodex, fulvestrant	Avoid high fat foods; exercise regularly to minimize possible weight gain side effect; eat foods rich in calcium and magnesium (dairy foods, broccoli, nuts and seeds). Avoid soy foods rich in phytoestrogens such as edamame, soy nuts and soy milk
Femara, letrozole	Avoid high fat foods; exercise regularly to minimize possible weight gain side effect; eat foods rich in calcium and magnesium (dairy foods, broccoli, nuts and seeds). Avoid soy foods rich in phytoestrogens such as edamame, soy nuts and soy milk
Fludara-IV, fludarabine	Drink extra fluids. Eat soft, bland foods
Folotyn, pralatrexate	Bland foods, avocado
Gemzar, gemcitabine	Drink extra fluids. If rash develops avoid foods high in salicylates (see list on page 11)
Gleevec, imatinib mesylate	Low sodium. Avoid grapefruit juice. Take with food
Gliadel, carmustine wafer	Drink extra fluids; restrict simple sugars
Halaven, eribulin mesylate	Drink extra fluids, high protein diet
Herceptin, trastuzumab	Bland diet. Flaxseed oil, extra virgin olive oil, walnuts and green tea may be beneficial. Grapefruit and curcumin should be avoided.
Hycamtin, topotecan	Include apple sauce, oatmeal and other soluble fiber rich foods to reduce diarrhea
Hydrea, hydroxyurea	Drink extra fluids
Idamycin, idarubicin	Drink extra fluids. Eat soft, moist foods.
Ifex, ifosfamide,	Drink extra fluids. Eat soft, moist foods
Iressa, gefitinib	Include apple sauce, oatmeal and other soluble fiber rich foods to reduce diarrhea. If rash develops avoid foods high in salicylates (see list on page 11)

Ixempra, ixabepilone	Maintain consistent diet. Eat soft, moist foods
Jevtana, cabazitaxel	Bland foods. Drink extra fluids. Extra protein
Leukeran, chlorambucil	Drink extra fluids; bland foods; avocado
Leukine, GM-CSF	Increase protein (add a whey protein smoothie)
Leustatin, cladribine	Include DHA. Extra protein
Lupron, leuprolide	Drink extra fluids. Eat diet high in vegetables and low in calories to prevent weight gain
Matulane, procarbazine	Avoid tyramine containing foods (aged cheeses, yogurt, raisins, eggplant, canned figs, salami, sour cream, avocados, bananas, soy sauce, lima beans, tenderized meats, etc. Ask for a list from your doctor) Maintain tyramine free diet for 14 days after treatment ceases; no alcohol
Mesnex, mesna	Take with strong flavored liquids like grape juice to avoid bad taste in mouth
Mustargen, mechlorethamine	Drink extra fluids; restrict simple sugars
Mutamycin, Mitomycin, MTC	Drink extra fluids; bland diet; avocado; eat foods rich in folate (green, leafy vegetables, citrus fruits) and foods rich in calcium (dairy foods, broccoli)
Mylocel, hydroxyurea	Drink extra fluids
Mylotarg, gemtuzumab, ozogamicin	Bland foods; avocado; Small, frequent meals
Navelbine, vinorelbine tartrate	Drink extra fluids
Neosar, cyclophosphamide	Drink extra fluids. Avoid alcohol; eat bland and low fat foods. Avoid turmeric and curcumin as it may interfere with drug effectiveness
Nexavar, sorafenib	Drink extra fluids. Banana, apple sauce, oatmeal if diarrhea occurs
Nilandron, nilutamide	Drink extra fluids
Nipent, pentostatin,	Bland foods; avocado. Small, frequent meals
Novantrone, mitoxantrone,	Drink extra fluids (discolored urine)
Oncovin, vincristine	Drink extra fluids; bland diet; avocado

Purinethol, mercaptopurine,	Drink extra fluids; avoid alcohol; avoid foods rich in purines (anchovies, kidneys, liver, meat extracts, sardines, beans and lentils) Eat foods rich in B vitamins like wheat germ
Revlimid, lenalidomide	Drink extra fluids. Include apple sauce, oatmeal and other soluble fiber rich foods to reduce diarrhea. If rash develops avoid foods high in salicylates (see list on page 14)
Roferon, interferon	Drink extra fluids; bland diet; avocado
Rituxan, rituximab	High fiber foods to prevent constipation. Use apple sauce and oatmeal if diarrhea occurs
Sandostatin, octreotide	Add lecithin granules (1 Tablespoon) to prevent possible gall stones if using long term
Sirolimus, rapamycin,	Avoid grapefruit and grapefruit juice which affects liver handling of this medication and may increase side effects
Sprycel, dasatinib	Avoid St John's Wort
Sutent, sunitinib	Avoid St John's Wort. Bland foods only. Avoid spicy foods, fatty foods and caffeine
Tamoxifen, nolvadex	Avoid high fat foods; exercise regularly to minimize possible weight gain side effect; eat foods rich in calcium and magnesium (dairy foods, broccoli, nuts and seeds). Avoid soy foods rich in phytoestrogens such as edamame, soy nuts and soy milk
Tarceva, erlotinib	Avoid spicy food. Soft diet
Targretin, bexarotene	Ensure sufficient iodine rich foods. Avoid grapefruit and grapefruit juice completely as it may interact with medication adversely
Tasigna, nilotinib	Avoid grapefruit juice. Take without food and wait one hour before eating
Taxol, paclitaxel	Avoid caffeine, avoid grapefruit juice. DHA may be helpful. Bland foods. Drink extra fluids. Extra protein (include a smoothie for example)
Taxotere, docetaxel	Avoid caffeine, avoid grapefruit juice. DHA may be helpful. Bland foods. Drink extra fluids. Extra protein (include a smoothie for example)
Temodar, temozolomide	Prevent possible constipation with high fiber foods, prune juice
TESPA. thiotepa	Extra protein, e.g. whey smoothie

Thalomid, thalidomide	Avoid alcohol which may increase sleepiness
TheraCys, BCG	Avoid caffeine and alcohol on treatment days
Thioguanine, 6-thioguanine	High fiber diet to prevent constipation
TICE, BCG	Avoid caffeine and alcohol on treatment days
Toposar, etoposide	Drink extra fluids. Try ginger for nausea. Bland diet. Soluble fiber rich foods (oatmeal, apple sauce) to prevent diarrhea
Torisel, temsirolimus,	Avoid St John's Wort. Apple sauce may help if diarrhea occurs
Treanda, bendamustine	High fiber foods to prevent constipation. Use apple sauce and oatmeal if diarrhea occurs
Trexall, methotrexate, mexate	Drink extra fluids; avoid alcohol; bland diet; eat foods that produce an alkaline urine to assist excretion (almonds, milk, fruits and vegetables, except cranberries, plums, corn and lentils)
Trisenox, arsenic trioxide	Try ginger to prevent nausea. Maintain consistent diet
Tykerb, lapatinib	Avoid grapefruit juice. Wait one hour before eating Maintain consistent fat content of diet
VCR, vincristine	Drink extra fluids; bland diet; avocado
Vesanoid, tretinoin, ATRA	Avoid vitamin A supplements. Add fiber to prevent constipation, e.g. wheat germ
Vectibix, panitumumab	High fiber diet to prevent constipation
Velban, vinblastine,	Drink extra fluids, no alcohol
Velcade, bortezomib, BZM	Avoid EGCG (green tea extract) supplements which block efficacy
VePesid, VP-16, etoposide	Bland foods; avocado
Viadur, leuprolide	Drink extra fluids. Eat diet high in vegetables and low in calories to prevent weight gain
Vidaza, azacitidine	Try ginger for nausea. Extra protein, e.g. whey
Vumon, teniposide	Drink extra fluids. Try ginger for nausea
Xeloda, capecitabine	Apple sauce, oatmeal and soluble fiber rich foods to prevent possible diarrhea
Zanosar, streptozocin	Drink extra fluids. Try ginger to avoid nausea
Zevalin, ibritumomab tiuxetan	Try ginger to avoid nausea

Zoladex, goserelin	Drink extra fluids. Low glycemic load (low sugar, high fiber) diet
Zometa, zoledronic acid	Drink extra fluids. Avoid calcium supplements

Drugs sometimes prescribed during treatment

Coumadin, warfarin	Maintain consistent intake of vitamin K rich foods (leafy green vegetables, liver) as these reduce effectiveness. No alcohol
Decadron, dexamethasone	Low salt, high potassium diet (avocado, bananas, citrus fruits, most vegetables)
Deltasone, prednisone	Low sugar diet. No alcohol
Epogen, epoetin alfa	Increase protein. Eggs (well cooked) may be helpful as they provide iron and protein
Intron A, interferon alpha	Increase protein, e.g. whey
Leukovorin, folinic acid	Given with 5-FU this is a form of the B vitamin folic acid that increases the activity of 5FU.
Megace, megestrol acetate	Low salt
Mesnex, mesna	Plenty of fluids
Meticorten, prednisone	Low salt
Neulasta, pegfilgrastim, G-CSF	Increase protein, e.g. whey
Neumega, oprevelkin, IL-11	Increase protein, e.g. whey
Neupogen, filgrastim	Increase protein, e.g. whey
Zinecard, dexrazoxane	Protects heart from Adriamycin potential side effects as a chelating agent. Ensure sufficient B vitamins and magnesium also

If your oncologist is using combinations of the above medications modify the advice so that you retain the most important parts. Remember to ask about nutrition; request a consultation with a Medical Nutrition Therapist (a registered dietitian or other qualified nutritionist).
Here is an example of dietary advice for a combination regimen:

CMF	Avoid fatty foods. Eat small quantities of bland flavors. Avoid alcohol, highly spiced foods or very acidic foods (cranberries, pineapple, lemons, etc.). Focus on vegetables, lean meats moistened in liquids such as stews, casseroles or in soups. Increase fiber with whole grain breakfast cereals

FOLFOX   Soft diet rich in soluble fiber like apple sauce to prevent diarrhea. Plenty of fluids. Avoid very cold foods or beverages with ice to minimize neuropathy

Many chemotherapy regimens affect your blood cell count. A nutritional supplement that is often described as hematinic, or blood building, may be valuable. Check with your oncologist before taking such a supplement in case it interferes with the chemotherapy. If you are prescribed a medication that stimulates new blood cell formation, include an extra serving of protein to get the optimal benefit. Remember to keep your health care team informed of all and any nutritional supplements (including herbal teas, fortified products and other functional foods).

RADIATION TREATMENT AND NUTRITION

Radiation may affect your taste buds so that food may taste bitter or you may have a metallic taste in your mouth. Some people find using non-metal utensils helpful. Try marinating meats for better flavor. Cold foods may be more palatable than hot but avoid extreme temperatures as your nerve endings may be compromised. Use herbs such as thyme, oregano, tarragon, mint and basil for added flavor. Try adding sauces such as apple sauce, yogurt dressings, mayonnaise and salad dressings to make food easier to chew. Snack on protein powder (whey, rice or soy) milk shakes. Ensure or other canned elemental diets are also useful standbys. Ask your health care professional or dietitian about products suitable for radiation enteritis or other chronic diarrhea situations. Examples include Resource Plus, Prosure, Vivonex and Peptamen. Radiation treatment should not be combined with high dose supplements of antioxidants (beta carotene, vitamins C and E or glutathione). The amounts found in a normal mixed diet will not interfere with treatment.
To counteract gastrointestinal problems avoid milk and milk products as lactose intolerance may develop. Yogurt which uses a live culture may be tolerated well. You can use Lactaid milk and Lactaid drops to minimize discomfort with dairy products. Ensure and similar meal replacement drinks are lactose free.

SOME SUPPLEMENTS AND HELPFUL FOODS

Alpha Lipoic Acid	An important antioxidant involved in detoxification
Coenzyme Q10	Another antioxidant that may be beneficial during treatment
Garlic	Allicin (allythio sulfinic allyl ester) is a weak anti-cancer agent found in garlic. Recognized as early as 1550 BC as a treatment for cancer.
Papaya, Guava or Pineapple	Many tropical fruits contain natural enzymes that may be beneficial during treatment and preventatively.
Green Tea	Contains protective botanical factors (catechins, polyphenols). Drink some daily.
Milk Thistle	This herb may assist in detoxification and general support of the liver detoxification enzyme systems. May be useful after chemotherapy. Also called Silymarin.

N-Acetyl Cysteine   Similar to alpha lipoic acid (see previous page), this is important in maintaining healthy liver and other tissue detoxification enzyme processes. Also called NAC.

Always consult with your physician before taking any nutritional supplements and inform all health care professionals of all supplements or medical foods you are taking regularly. Make a list and share it with everyone even if you think they don't understand or support you. *This is very important.*

SOME IMPORTANT REMINDERS

1. Do not take any additional antioxidants for one day before and at least two days after any treatment to optimize treatment. Antioxidants may interfere with the clearance of some chemotherapy agents. Some oncologists prefer that you stop all supplements except milk thistle for the three days around treatment.

2. Eat small amounts of food every few hours rather than big meals. You may find your appetite is best in the morning; this is a good time to eat a healthy breakfast. Don't go for longer than eight hours overnight without something with calories as this is when your body needs energy the most. Try sipping papaya or apricot nectar or pineapple juice if you wake up as these are easy to digest. Rinse right afterwards with water.

3. Drink plenty of fluids; use water, clear soups and juices in preference to caffeinated beverages. Rinse with lightly salted water if your mouth is sore.

4. Imagine your digestion as that of a young child. Eat only small quantities at a time of easy to digest foods. Small jars of weaning baby food may be helpful as ready-to-eat supplemental snack meals. Protein smoothies are useful to sip on. Try garnishing them with fresh fruit to make them more appealing.

5. Microwave or moist cook fruits and vegetables to improve their digestibility.

6. If fruit upsets your stomach, try tropical juices instead. You can also dilute with water.

7. Experiment with different foods in small amounts. Everyone's digestion is unique. Some people find spicy foods helpful while others do not.

Remember we are all different. There is no right or wrong way to eat. Staying healthy and strong is what is important.

HERBS AND SURGERY WARNINGS

The American Medical Association recently issued the following warnings about herbs that should be discontinued prior to surgery:

Herb	Discontinue Period Prior to Surgery
Ephedra	At least 24 hours before surgery
Garlic	At least 7 days before surgery
Ginkgo	At least 36 hours before surgery
Ginseng	At least 7 days before surgery
Kava	At least 24 hours before surgery
St. John's Wort	At least 5 days before surgery
Valerian	Taper off several weeks before surgery. Suddenly stopping can cause withdrawal problems.

Source:
Use of Herbal Medications before Surgery. Betz et al. JAMA.2001; 286: 2542-2544.
TELL YOUR MEDICAL TEAM ABOUT ANY SUPPLEMENTS YOU ARE TAKING.

FOODS FOR HEALTH

Every day you consume some 23,000 different chemicals. Most of these chemicals need to be metabolized before excretion and in order to protect from potential toxicity or damage we need to eat foods regularly that support this complex system of enzymes. Foods rich in the 3 A's (Antioxidants, Anti-inflammatories and Anticarcinogens) may be helpful in promoting healthy liver function and support of immune health. They include the following:

- Acorn squash
- Asparagus
- Avocado
- Bitter melon
- Blackberries
- Black currants
- Black raspberries
- Blueberries
- Broccoli
- Cabbage
- Cantaloupe
- Cruciferous vegetable family
- Garlic
- Grapes
- Green tea
- Orange (especially the zest from the rind)
- Pomegranates
- Potatoes
- Parsley
- Pistachios
- Red raspberries
- Spinach
- Strawberries
- Tomatoes
- Turmeric
- Walnuts
- Watercress
- Zucchini

Suggested Supplements

Multivitamin and mineral	Centrum, Blue Bonnet Multi-One capsules or Solgar's Univite or Designs for Health
Alpha Lipoic Acid	60 milligrams daily
Coenzyme Q10	120 milligrams daily
Selenium	200 micrograms daily
Vitamin E (as mixed tocopherols)	200 IU daily

During treatment (optional and only with oncologist approval)

Astragalus root	1 capsule (Solgar)
Milk thistle (Silymarin)	80 milligrams (Solgar)

SUGGESTIONS FOR HANDLING TREATMENT SIDE EFFECTS

Eating well is vital to give you that extra edge as you participate in your own recovery. Choose healthy foods to empower yourself for this important time in your life. Each time you choose a fruit, vegetable or protein rich food you are giving your body what it needs to fight the cancer. Improved nutrition can also help you to withstand the side effects of chemotherapy, radiation and surgery. Some treatments may make eating difficult or distasteful but there are many valuable medications available to minimize side effects. Remember to ask ahead so you can prevent rather than treat nausea, diarrhea and constipation.

Here are some specific nutrition suggestions to help you with some of the most common treatment-related problems. Even if some of these ideas appear to be in conflict with the basic high fiber/low saturated animal fat concepts you are familiar with, maintaining a reasonably constant body weight is your overriding priority at this time. Choose fats or oils that contain more of the beneficial fatty acids to boost calories as well as support your immunity. Examples include olives (and olive oil), avocados, nuts (almonds, walnuts and Brazil nuts are particularly good - nut butters are valuable ways of consuming them) and seeds (sunflower or pumpkin).

Suggestions for chewing and swallowing difficulties:
1. Eat foods prepared with moist heat such as soups, stews, casseroles or pasta
2. Add gravy, sauces, butter, mayonnaise or salad dressings to make food easier to swallow
3. Avoid highly seasoned, spicy, tart or acidic foods such as tomatoes
4. Avoid alcohol and smoking
5. Cold foods may be soothing if there are sores in the mouth. Use a straw. Ice chips or popsicles may be helpful
6. Keep your caloric intake high by using protein smoothies and meal replacement drinks (ready-to-drink, e.g. Boost® or Muscle Milk®)
7. If you have trouble swallowing soups, try using a cup or glass instead of a spoon. Texture may become especially important
8. Try carbonated drinks as they may be easier to swallow. Carbonation often helps with nausea by releasing upper gas. Try ginger ale as ginger is also good for preventing nausea

Suggestions for dealing with diarrhea:

1. Choose oatmeal, white rice and other refined grain products
2. Chicken noodle soup is an old standby; home made is best
3. Avoid eating raw fruits and vegetables except bananas. Peel all vegetables before cooking and remove skins and seeds. Avoid nuts unless in butter form, e.g. almond butter. No popcorn
4. Avoid high fiber foods that contain a great deal of roughage; for instance wheat bran, wheat germ or whole wheat. Ice berg lettuce, onions, garlic, cucumber and celery may also cause intestinal distress. Avoid harsh textured foods
5. Eat cooked apples, apple sauce or apple puree. This is binding
6. Don't drink more than 1 cup of fluid with your meals, but drink plenty of water in between
7. Eat frequent, small meals rather than three large ones
8. Food and liquids should be warm or at room temperature, rather than very hot or ice cold
9. If the diarrhea is severe, restrict your diet to clear liquids such as broth, flat ginger ale, tea or sports types of drinks (Gatorade or PowerAde) for one day. If it persists for more than one day, call your physician

Suggestions for dealing with constipation:

1. Drink plenty of fluids. At least 1 liter of water daily
2. Eat prunes, apricots, peaches, cherries or other pitted fruit
3. Drink prune juice
4. Use syrup of figs as a gentle laxative
5. Eat rhubarb (only the red parts, stewed)
6. Add wheat bran or wheat germ or ground flaxseed on top of cereal
7. Exercise, stretching and all types of movements help stimulate the circulation which may ease constipation. Avoid sitting for long periods to avoid hemorrhoids
8. Maintain a regular morning schedule allowing plenty of time
9. Try a hot drink and then relax. Avoid straining

Suggestions for dealing with nausea and/or vomiting:

1. Eat and drink slowly
2. Eat small, frequent meals, chewed well
3. Try ginger ale or crystallized ginger
4. Avoid greasy, fatty and fried foods
5. Rest after meals
6. For early morning or pre-meal nausea, try a cracker or dry toast
7. Make up for lost calories when you feel more comfortable
8. Avoid cooking odors by microwaving. Use a fan in the kitchen
9. Try crushed ice types of drinks

Suggestions for loss of appetite:

1. If you aren't hungry at dinnertime, make breakfast or lunch your main meal. Similarly, if you aren't hungry first thing in the morning, eat more later
2. Eat more frequently, but smaller amounts of food
3. Keep snacks readily available, e.g. in your purse or in the car
4. Always make food look attractive with garnishes or with place settings
5. Experiment with tastes - you may find things you didn't like before, you like now. Umami found in Asian food is often a taste that appeals when the other 4 receptor cell types are affected; salty, sweet, bitter or sour. Try some miso soup for example as an appetizer
6. Cold or room temperature foods may be more appealing
7. A glass of wine or beer may increase your appetite (check with your doctor first in case alcohol doesn't mix with a medication)
8. Increase the caloric intake of the foods that you do eat with a small amount of "light" (less strongly flavored, not fewer calories) olive oil
9. Try a protein smoothie or one of the commercially prepared meal replacement drinks such as Boost®. Whey protein powder is easy to digest and nutritious

Please visit my website at www.cancernutrition.com for more suggestions.

SUGGESTIONS FOR EATING TO PROVIDE MAXIMUM IMMUNITY

By making wise eating choices, you may be able to fortify your natural defenses and handle treatments with ease. Remember to take extra care with personal hygiene such as having regular manicures and pedicures, taking care to wash your hands frequently at this time as your immune system may be compromised due to treatment. Listen to your body's needs for rest and sleep. You will benefit from being in natural surroundings and by keeping the company of those who don't drain you of energy.

As each person's nutritional needs are very individual, I suggest that you see a nutritionist or Registered Dietitian (RD) at this time to assist you in making healthy food choices. Make a weekly food and exercise diary and place it on the refrigerator. This way you can monitor your changes in a way that is valuable for you, your family and your health care team.

The following essential nutrients maintain healthy immunity

Nutrient	Food Source
Vitamin A	Fish liver oils, liver
Beta Carotene (Pro-vitamin A)	Orange, yellow and dark green vegetables including carrots, cantaloupe, apricots and spinach

Nutrient	Food Source
Vitamin B1 (Thiamin)	Whole grains, fortified breakfast cereals
Vitamin B2 (Riboflavin)	Whole and enriched cereal and breads, lean meat, milk, eggs and organic calf or lamb liver
Vitamin B3 (Niacin)	Whole grains, eggs, liver
Vitamin B6 (Pyridoxine)	Whole grains, lean meat, eggs, organic calf or lamb liver
Folic acid	Whole grains, leafy vegetables, meat
Pantothenic acid	Brewer's yeast, beans, salmon
Vitamin C	Citrus fruits, kiwi, strawberries, peppers
Vitamin D	Oily fish, fortified foods (milk, etc.)
Vitamin E	Egg yolk, liver, wheat germ, nuts, and seeds
Iron	Peas, liver, egg yolk, asparagus
Lycopene	Pink grapefruit, guava, tomatoes
Magnesium	Leafy vegetables, nuts, seafood
Manganese	Bananas, bran, pineapple, nuts
Selenium	Garlic, legumes, fish, asparagus
Sulfur	Garlic, avocado, lean meat
Zinc	Oysters, liver, sunflower seeds
Phytochemicals	Dark pigmented herbs, berries
Antioxidants	Blueberries, cocoa, red grapes, kiwi, culinary herbs
Protein	Eggs, lean meat, poultry, fish, shellfish, tofu, beans and rice

SUGAR

Does sugar feed cancer? This question is the most common one I receive on my website www.cancernutrition.com The answer is not a simple one as we are all different and cancer itself is not one disease but a multitude of different genetic mutations. If you have a glucose sensitive metabolism or if your particular cancer has resulted in changes in glucose sensitivity then sugar may be feeding your cancer and we recommend that you reduce your intake to less than 30 grams per day or not exceeding 15 grams per meal or per drink. This won't harm anyone but is particularly important for some people.

Most cancer cells develop the capacity to use energy from glucose (one of the two components of table sugar or sucrose) without needing oxygen. This means that the cells are able to survive when most other cells cannot. We can't live without glucose or oxygen however. We need both for all of our healthy cells.

Please see my website www.cancernutrition.com for an article on sugar that is more extensive.

INFLAMMATORY PROCESSES AND CANCER

Inflammation is thought to play a critical role in cancer processes. Anti-inflammatory foods are important for everyone and are especially important for those dealing with cancer. Anti-inflammatory foods fight inflammatory processes.

Omega-3 oils are important anti-inflammatory foods and are found in blue-green algae and spirulina. Ocean fish consume these tiny plant-like substances and concentrate them and thus the fish then become excellent sources of omega-3 oils. Krill oil is also an excellent source of omega-3 fatty acids. Salmon, herrings and sardines are some of the richest sources of these important oils that enhance anti-inflammatory processes in the body.

Omega-3 oils are important in all nervous system functions. A panel of nutritionists and scientists at the National Institutes of Health recently recommended that a ratio of omega-6 (thought to be pro-inflammatory) to omega-3 (anti-inflammatory) oils should ideally be 4. The usual dietary intake in the United States is currently about 10-20:1 omega-6: omega-3. The best way to adjust the ratio is to cut down on omega-6 and include more omega-3 rich foods such as salmon, pine nuts and walnuts. You may also wish to include a supplement of EPA and DHA (the principle omega-3 oils). Algae are now used to manufacture omega-3 that doesn't have an aftertaste and is used to fortify foods including milk.

Omega-3 oils are found in oily fish, nuts such as walnuts, macadamia, pecans and certain seeds and vegetables. GLA (Gamma linoleic acid) is an important oil found in flaxseed. Evening primrose, black currant seed and borage are other supplemental sources. GLA is good for regulating hormone and prostaglandins (short acting local hormones). GLA may be taken as a supplement.

Anti-inflammatory processes are favored when you balance your oils and fats:
    Choose oily fish, nuts and seeds often
    Watch your intake of cheese, butter and bacon
    Use cold pressed extra virgin olive oil in salad dressings
    Sprinkle pine nuts on salads
    Choose avocado often

Other sources of Anti-inflammatory nutrients
Many vegetables are also rich in anti-inflammatory aspirin like substances also called COX-

inhibitors. Examples include apricots, broccoli, turmeric, raspberries, loganberries, pineapple, curry, rosemary, thyme and tarragon.

Choose foods that have properties that are the 3 A's - Antioxidants, Anti-inflammatories and Anticarcinogens

DIGESTIVE ENZYMES

What are digestive enzymes?
Digestive enzymes are proteins that assist in the digestion of food. These proteins catalyze the breaking down of nutrients into more absorbable forms.
> Proteases help break down proteins
> Amylases help break down carbohydrates (starches)
> Lactase helps with lactose digestion
> Lipases help break down fats and oils

Do I need to take an enzyme supplement?
Some people benefit from taking supplemental digestive enzymes especially during chemotherapy or after radiation to the digestive tract region. Digestive enzymes can reduce abdominal discomfort and gas. Wobenzyme-N is a good example of a high quality digestive enzyme supplement containing Bromelain (from pineapple) and papain (from papaya).

Which foods contain digestive enzymes?
Pineapple, papaya and guava are good sources of proteases.

Are these supplements safe to take?
Yes, these are safe supplements and may enhance white cell activity which is often helpful during chemotherapy.

IF SOMEONE YOU LOVE HAS CANCER

Learning that someone you love has cancer may be one of the most frightening moments of your life. This is often because of the things we have heard or read that make it sound like a death sentence. However, this simply isn't true. Today there are more than 10 million cancer survivors in America and for most people who are diagnosed with cancer; it will not be the reason for their death. Heart disease is the leading cause of death for the age group that is most affected by cancer. One of the most important things you can do for yourself and for your loved one is to find out exactly what the facts are about their diagnosis. The American Cancer Society is the most respected and trusted source of cancer information and they can be reached 24 hours a day (toll free) at 1-800-4CANCER or on their website www.cancer.org.

I encourage you to gather relevant paperwork such as copies of biopsy and blood test results and keep them in a folder. Write down questions to ask the medical professionals and write down the answers received. Many people find that keeping records lowers their anxiety level and gives them a feeling of control. Typical questions might be:

    What is my diagnosis? What stage is my cancer at?
    How aggressive is the cancer?
    How long will I receive treatment for?
    How will I feel after my treatments?
    Is there anything I should avoid?
    Can I continue to exercise?
    Are there foods I should avoid?
    Is the treatment likely to make me nauseous?
    Is the treatment likely to give me diarrhea/constipation?
    Are there over the counter medications I should have on hand?
    How will I know how I am progressing?
    How often will I have scans/blood tests?
    Is there a clinical trial I am eligible for?

SAMPLE FOOD CHOICES

Breakfast choices
    Whole grain type of dry cereal
    Eggs (poached, scrambled, boiled or as an omelet)
    Oatmeal or other hot cereal
    Whole grain bread, toast or bagel

Snack
    Fresh fruit
    Small protein smoothie (4-6 fluid ounces)
    Greek style yogurt

Lunch
    Ginger-sesame salmon
    Brown rice
    Asparagus spears
    topped with slivered almonds
    OR
    Chicken breast and walnuts
    Garlic mashed potatoes
    Red cabbage
    OR

Lunch, cont.
    Bean, noodle and nut deep dish
    Salad of leafy, young dark greens
    topped with Balsamic vinegar and extra virgin olive oil salad dressing
    OR
    Vegetable curry
    Brown rice
    Fruit chutney
    OR
    Lentil and pecan deep dish
    Grated carrots, beets and radish salad
    Olive oil and rice vinegar salad dressing
    OR
    White fish with fresh ginger and lemon
    Brown rice
    Spinach with olive oil and garlic
    OR
    Frittata with spinach
    Tomato and Maui onion salad
    Extra virgin olive oil and pine nuts

Snack
- Small handful of dried apricot and almonds
- Ginger snap cookie and milk

Dinner
- Pasta primavera
- Asparagus tips garnish
- Small side salad

OR

- Stir-fry vegetables on bed of brown rice

OR

- Tasty rice and tofu
- Spinach salad with slivered almonds
- Olive oil and balsamic vinegar dressing

OR

- Halibut with broccoli and almonds
- Brown rice
- Sliced buffalo tomatoes

OR

Dinner, cont.
- Sea bass with apples
- Mashed potatoes
- Brussels sprouts and chestnuts
- Cherry tomatoes

OR

- Teriyaki salmon
- Fingerling potatoes
- Broccolini (steamed)
- Garlic and parsley butter topping

OR

- Risotto
- Salad of mixed dark leafy greens
- Olive oil and balsamic vinegar dressing

Desserts and comfort foods
- Fruit Brown Betty
- Egg custard
- Ice cream (made with high quality ingredients)

When selecting your or a loved one's menu plans remember that taste buds may be affected by the treatment. Adjust seasonings accordingly and avoid strong flavors that may irritate mouth and gums. Create an environment that is as stress free as possible; add flowers to your table or tray setting, avoid challenging conversations or other upsetting distractions. Many people enjoy eating in restaurants because they don't have to choose what to eat hours ahead, someone else cleans up and the environment is usually quiet and supportive.

It is also a good idea to eat the most in the morning or at midday. Our bodies have a natural circadian rhythm that encourages us to eat earlier in the day so we can move around and digest best. Eating a lot in the evening isn't recommended as it may interfere with restful sleep.

SOME DIET SUGGESTIONS

To increase calories

Add avocado to salads or sandwiches. Slice in half and squeeze fresh lemon or lime juice, twisting the rind to extract essential oils such as limonene which are important at inducing apoptosis (programmed cell death). Add olive or hazelnut oil to vegetables

Be generous with salad dressings

To increase protein
- Add protein powder to fruit juices and smoothies
- Include cottage cheese often
- Include Greek style yogurt often
- Add hard boiled eggs and egg whites to salads
- Add skim dry milk powder to recipes

To increase cancer fighting phytonutrients or botanical factors
- Choose asparagus often
- Drink pomegranate juice (1-2 fluid ounces daily)
- Choose curry, cook with turmeric and cumin
- Choose blueberries, raspberries and cranberries often
- Choose rhubarb

To increase iron
- Choose peas
- Choose eggs (yolk is rich in iron)
- Choose asparagus
- Choose lean red meat
- Choose organic lamb or chicken liver

To increase magnesium
- Choose lean red meat, dark meat poultry, liver, shellfish, oysters
- Choose fortified breakfast cereals, enriched bread, oatmeal
- Choose sunflower seeds

To increase zinc
- Choose dark green leafy vegetables
- Choose nuts and nut butters
- Choose oysters and shellfish

For general blood building properties
- Choose organic liver or liver sausage
- Prepare soups with marrow bone broth (see recipe)
- Choose osso buco and other marrow bone recipes

Each time you select a food with additional benefits you are making a positive health move. This is empowering and your body will thank you.

MY DAILY FOOD GUIDE

Food I choose to eat   Liquids   How I feel   Notes

Summary of the Day

Appetite: Fluids: Other information:

Make as many copies of this page as you need and post on the refrigerator for your health team members to help assist you in providing the care you need.

HELPFUL RECIPES

If your mouth is sore:

Babaghanoush	33
Chicken and Okra Gumbo	41
Green Pea Soup	44
Root Vegetable Soup	50
Brown Rice Pilaf	56
Risotto	67
Spaghetti with Artichoke Hearts	68
Tasty Rice and Tofu	71
Creamy Dijon Sole	76
Garlic Mashed Potatoes	98
Angel Food Cake	109
Key Lime Pie	115
Apple Pie Smoothie	125
Banana Fruit Smoothie	126
Black Forest Smoothie	127
Cappuccino Smoothie	128
Extra Chocolatey Smoothie	129
Passionate Papaya Smoothie	134
Peach Milk Smoothie	135
Soda Fountain Shake	138
Vanilla Smoothie	142

If you are constipated:

Bean Dip	34
Guacamole	38
Chicken Soup	42
Gazpacho	43
Green Pea Soup	44
Immuno-Soup	45
Minestrone	46
Phytomineral Soup	48
Root Vegetable	50
Adzuki Beans and Rice	52
Baked Beans	53
Bean, Noodle and Nut Casserole	54
Blackeyed Peas	55
Flageolets	57
Lentil and Pecan Casserole	59
Lentil Patties	60
Mexican Bean Pie	61

If you are constipated, cont.:

Navy Bean Stew	62
Pasta Primavera	65
Quinoa-Nut Vegetable Pilaf	66
Spaghetti with Artichoke Hearts	68
Southern Style Beans and Rice	69
Tasty Rice and Tofu	71
Broiled Orange Roughy	75
Monkfish, Mushrooms and Lentils	80
Sea Bass with Apples	81
White Fish with Ginger and Lemon	85
Brussels Sprouts and Chestnuts	91
Eggplant Parmesan	94
French Peas	96
Spinach, Brown Rice and Tofu	103
Sweet and Sour Vegetables	104
Vegetable Curry	106
Vegetarian Stew	107
Apricot and Strawberry Cake	111
Ginger Cookies	113
Fresh Fruit Salad	119
Pears in Red Wine	121
Apple Pie Smoothie	125
Banana Fruit Smoothie	126
Black Forest Smoothie	127
Extra Chocolatey Smoothie	129
Passionate Papaya Smoothie	134
Prune Smoothie	136
Raspberry RazMaTaz	137
Strawberry Daiquiri	140
Strawberry Sensation	141

If you have diarrhea:

Miso soup	47
Cinnamon Apple Sauce	117

If your white cell count is low:

Chicken Liver Pâté	36
Beef broth	39
Chicken broth	40

APPETIZERS

Babaghanoush

- 2 medium eggplants
- 1 pinch cumin powder
- 1 tablespoon lemon juice
- 1 ½ tablespoons nonfat yogurt
- 1 tablespoon tahini
- 1 clove garlic, crushed
- 2 tablespoons fresh parsley, chopped

Bake the eggplant in a medium oven until cooked through (about 20 minutes). Remove the skin and place in a blender. Add the tahini, yogurt, garlic, lemon juice and cumin powder. Blend to desired consistency. Season to taste and chill before serving. Garnish with chopped parsley.

Note: Good source of folic acid

Serves 4
Prep Time: 0:25

Calories 90	Carbohydrate 16g	Cholesterol 0gm
Protein 4g	Fat 2g	Dietary Fiber 3g
	% Calories from fat 22%	

APPETIZERS

Bean Dip

- ½ cup beans, soaked overnight
- 1 tablespoon fresh chives, chopped
- ½ tablespoon extra virgin olive oil
- ¼ teaspoon salt
- 2 tablespoons salsa
- ¼ teaspoon black pepper

Rinse and drain the beans (any type is good). Boil for 20 minutes or until tender. If using canned beans, drain. Transfer to a blender and blend until smooth. Add the salsa, oil, salt and black pepper and continue to blend. Place in a serving bowl and chill. Serve with blue corn chips as an appetizer.

Notes: Excellent source of Folic acid. Good source of Vitamin B1. You can use the recipe for Salsa or purchase ready mixed salsa. Canned beans may also be used.

Serves: 5
Prep Time: 0:30

Calories	106	Carbohydrate 16g	Cholesterol 0mg
Protein	6g	Fat 2g	Dietary Fiber 6g
		% Calories from fat 19%	

Bruschetta

- 4 slices Italian bread
- 4 plum tomatoes, sliced
- 2 garlic cloves
- 2 tablespoons fresh basil, chopped
- ½ tablespoon olive oil
- ½ teaspoon black pepper, fresh ground

Use a broiler to toast the bread on both sides. Rub the upper surfaces with garlic and sprinkle with olive oil. Top with slices of tomato and sprinkle with fresh basil and black pepper. Serve immediately while the toast is still warm.

Notes: Excellent source of Vitamin C and lycopene. Good source of Vitamin A, B1, B2, Folate and Niacin.

Serves: 4
Prep Time: 0:15

Calories 123	Carbohydrate 21g	Cholesterol 0mg
Protein 4g	Fat 3g	Dietary Fiber 2g
	% Calories from fat 22%	

APPETIZERS

Chicken Liver Pâté

- ¾ pound chicken livers
- 2 egg whites, hard boiled
- ½ medium Spanish onion
- ¼ teaspoon salt
- 1 stalk celery, finely chopped
- ½ teaspoon black pepper
- ¼ green bell pepper, finely chopped
- 1 teaspoon olive oil

In a non stick skillet sprayed with olive oil, gently sauté the chicken livers for 2-3 minutes until firm but not completely cooked through. Place the livers and hard boiled egg whites together in a blender and blend until smooth. Add the celery and green bell pepper and combine by hand with the seasonings. Place in a pâté dish or small soufflé dish and chill in the refrigerator. A thin layer of clarified butter on top will keep the pâté fresh for a few days in the refrigerator. Serve garnished with a little chopped parsley and with triangles of thinly sliced toast.

Notes: Excellent source of Vitamin C, A, B6, B12, B2, Folate, Niacin and Iron. Good source of Zinc.

If you like pâté, this is a lower fat, lower cholesterol version that still retains good flavor. Liver pâté is a nutritious appetizer.

Serves: 6
Prep Time: 0:05
Stand Time: 0:30

Calories 90	Carbohydrate 4 g	Cholesterol 249 mg
Protein 12g	Fat 3g	Dietary Fiber 0g
	% Calories from fat 30%	

APPETIZERS

Curry Dip

- ⅓ cup plain low fat yogurt
- 2 drops Tabasco sauce
- 2 teaspoons curry powder
- ¼ teaspoon black pepper
- 1 teaspoon fresh lemon juice
- 1 teaspoon sugar

Combine the ingredients together and place in a serving dish. Garnish with cayenne or paprika. Serve with crackers and fresh vegetables.

Notes: Good source of Vitamin C.

Serves: 4
Prep Time: 0:05

Calories 20	Carbohydrate 3g	Cholesterol 1mg
Protein 1g	Fat 2g	Dietary Fiber 0g
	% Calories from fat 18%	

APPETIZERS

Guacamole

- 2 avocados
- 1 green bell pepper, peeled and chopped
- ¼ cup fresh lemon juice
- 1 fresh cilantro, finely chopped
- 1 clove garlic, crushed
- ½ teaspoon salt
- 6 tomatoes, peeled and chopped
- ¼ teaspoon black pepper
- 1 medium onion, chopped

Peel, remove the pit and mash the avocado. Add the lemon juice, garlic, tomatoes, onion and pepper. Stir in the cilantro. Replace the avocado pit to keep the guacamole from turning brown. Serve with corn chips.

Notes: Excellent source of Vitamin C, A, B6, Folate. Good source of Vitamin B1, B2, Niacin and Iron.

Eat sparingly as this is a high-fat food. Fat content is of good fatty acid profile and this dish is a good source of antioxidants.

Serves: 4
Prep Time: 0:10

Calories 214	Carbohydrate 19g	Cholesterol 0mg
Protein 4g	Fat 16g	Dietary Fiber 5g
		% Calories from fat 60%

SOUPS

The foundation of most soups is a good broth. Here are some examples of broths that provide blood building factors as well as taste.

Beef (or veal) Stock

    1 teaspoon olive oil
    2 pounds of beef with bones in
    (such as rib or long bones cut by the butcher into 3-inch pieces)
    4 cups water
    ½ teaspoon salt
    1 clove garlic
    1 onion, diced
    1 carrot, diced
    1 stalk celery, diced
    12 peppercorns
    Bouquet garni (dried thyme, rosemary, and oregano in a muslin bag)

Heat the oil in a large, heavy saucepan and quickly fry the bones to provide flavor. Cover the bones with the water, add the salt, and bring to a boil. Skim the froth off the top and discard; add the vegetables and the peppercorns. Boil slowly for 4 to 5 hours. Strain the liquid with a fine sieve and use immediately as a soup base. The bones may be used with fresh vegetables up to two more times and still provide healthful nutrients.

SOUPS

Chicken Stock

1	whole chicken, cut into pieces
8	cups water
2	small carrots, chopped
1	stalk celery, chopped
1	onion, chopped

Place all the ingredients in a large pot. Bring to a boil, then reduce the heat to low. Cook for 2 hours, skimming the froth and the oil every 20 to 30 minutes; discard. Remove the meat and the vegetables and serve separately as a main dish with mashed potatoes, pasta, or rice. Strain the liquid broth to use as a base for other soups or clarified as chicken consommé.

Clarified Broth

Clarification of both chicken and beef stock is done after the broth is first passed through a cheesecloth or very fine sieve and all visible particles have been removed. Combine ¼ cup cold water with one egg white and crushed eggshell. Bring to a boil, then remove from heat and allow to stand for 5 minutes. Strain again to produce a clear liquid, also called consommé.

SOUPS

Chicken and Okra Gumbo

- 2 chicken breast halves, skinless
- 4 garlic cloves, crushed
- 2 tablespoons olive oil
- 1 tablespoon Worcestershire sauce
- 2 cups chopped okra
- 1½ teaspoon Creole seasoning
- 1 medium chopped onion
- ½ cup cooked rice
- 2 sticks chopped celery
- 2 quarts water
- 1 medium chopped green bell pepper
- 1 can (15 ounces) tomatoes
- ¼ teaspoon filé (optional)
- 1 ounce chopped scallions

Heat half of the oil in a heavy-bottomed casserole dish. Dust the chicken with flour and brown for 4-6 minutes on each side. Remove and set aside in a warm place. Add the rest of the oil and sauté the okra for 10 minutes stirring constantly. Add the onion, celery, bell pepper and garlic and continue to cook for 1-2 minutes. Add the chicken, tomatoes, Worcestershire sauce, seasonings and water and bring to a boil. Reduce the heat, cover the pan and simmer for 2 hours or until the chicken is tender. Skim excess fat and serve with rice in soup bowls. Garnish with chopped scallions and a sprinkling of filé, if available.

Notes: Excellent source of Vitamin C, B6 and Folate
Good source of Vitamin A, B1 and Niacin.

Serving Size: 4
Prep Time: 0:20
Cooking Time: 2:00

Calories 276	Carbohydrate 30g	Cholesterol 33mg
Protein 17g	Fat 11g	Dietary Fiber 5g
	% Calories from fat 35%	

SOUPS

Chicken Soup

- 3 pounds chicken, skinless light meat cut in pieces
- 4 quarts water
- 3 stalks chopped celery
- 2 bay leaves
- 1 medium chopped onion
- ½ teaspoon pepper
- 2 sliced leeks
- 1 teaspoon paprika
- 2 sprigs parsley
- 3 cloves crushed garlic
- ½ tablespoon olive oil
- 3 medium sliced carrots

Heat the oil in a large, heavy based pan. Sauté the onions and garlic for 3-4 minutes. Add the water, paprika, salt, pepper and bay leaves. Bring to a boil, cover and simmer for 2 hours. Remove from the heat, cut the chicken into small pieces and remove the bones. Return the chicken to the pan and add the carrots, celery, onions and parsley. Simmer for another hour. Serve hot.

Notes: Excellent source of Vitamin C, A, B6, B12, B2, Niacin, Calcium, Iron and Zinc. Good source of Vitamin B1 and Folate.

Serving Size: 4
Prep Time: 0:10
Cooking Time: 3:00

Calories 332	Carbohydrate 25g	Cholesterol 99mg
Protein 48g	Fat 6g	Dietary Fiber 6g
	% Calories from fat 16%	

Gazpacho

- 1 clove crushed garlic
- 2 cups tomato juice
- 6 cups chopped tomatoes
- ½ teaspoon cumin
- 1 medium chopped onion
- ½ teaspoon ground black pepper
- ½ cup chopped green pepper
- ½ teaspoon salt
- ½ cup chopped cucumber
- 1 tablespoon extra virgin olive oil
- ¼ cup fine ground breadcrumbs
- ¼ cup fresh lemon juice

Blend the tomatoes, garlic, onion and green pepper in a blender. Add the cucumber and strain into a serving bowl containing the breadcrumbs. Mix well and chill for 30 minutes in the refrigerator. Before serving, blend the olive oil, lemon juice, salt, pepper, cumin and tomato juice. Stir into the mixture and serve garnished with small dishes of diced tomatoes, cucumber and green pepper.

Notes: Excellent source of Vitamin A, C, B6 and Folate. Good source of Calcium.

Serving Size: 6
Prep Time: 0:10
Stand Time: 0:30

Calories 112	Carbohydrate 20g	Cholesterol 0mg
Protein 4g	Fat 3g	Dietary Fiber 4g
	% Calories from fat 23%	

SOUPS

Green Pea Soup

- ½ tablespoon olive oil
- 1 teaspoon oregano
- 2 medium chopped onions
- ½ teaspoon black pepper
- 1 stalks chopped celery
- ½ teaspoon salt
- 1 ½ cups split peas
- ½ teaspoon dry mustard
- 4 cups water

Soak the split peas overnight and drain the water. Heat the oil in a saucepan and sauté the onions and celery for 3-4 minutes. Add the celery and cook for another 2 minutes. Add the water and peas and bring to a boil. Cover and simmer for 20 minutes or until the peas become mushy. Place in the blender or in a food processor with a metal blade to blend. Add oregano and adjust seasoning. Serve hot with croutons.

Notes: Excellent source of Vitamin B1 and Folate. Good source of Vitamin B6, Iron and Zinc.

Serving Size: 6
Prep Time: 0:30 (overnight for soaking of split peas)

Calories 192	Carbohydrate 33	Cholesterol 0g
Protein 13g	Fat 2g	Dietary Fiber 14g
	% Calories from fat 8%	

Immuno-Soup

1 cup beans soaked overnight or canned	½ teaspoon orega[no]
2 whole carrots, sliced thin	½ pounds sliced gr[een beans]
1 whole rutabaga, chopped	½ teaspoon marjora[m]
1 whole beet, sliced	4 whole zucchini, sliced thin
1 whole turnip, chopped	½ teaspoon rosemary
1 whole potato, diced	1 bunch scallions, sliced
2 cloves crushed garlic	½ teaspoon sage
1 head celery, chopped	1 pound spinach, chopped
½ bell pepper, chopped	1 teaspoon thyme
1 bunch parsley, chopped	½ head cauliflower, broken in pieces

Soak beans overnight and discard water. Wash and prepare the vegetables. Place the root vegetables (carrots, potatoes, turnip, parsnip or rutabaga) into a large pot with the beans. Half fill the pot with water and bring to a boil. Cover and simmer for 10 minutes. Add all of the other ingredients and season to taste. Return to a boil and cook uncovered for 1-2 minutes more. Cover and simmer for another 30 minutes. Adjust seasoning and serve hot or cold.

This soup improves with age. Split into 1-2 cup-sized servings and freeze for a quick and healthy meal. You can add grated cheese to the surface of a bowl and melt it under a hot grill. For variety include brown rice, barley, noodles or corn. Tamari, soy sauce or Bragg's liquid aminos also add flavor.

Notes: Excellent source of Vitamin C, A, B6, B1, B2, Folate, Calcium and Iron. Good source of Niacin and Zinc.

Serving Idea: Serve with hot crusty bread.

Serving Size: 8
Prep Time: 0:45

Calories 179	Carbohydrate 35g	Cholesterol 0mg
Protein 12g	Fat 1g	Dietary Fiber 13g
	% Calories from fat 5%	

Minestrone

- 1 cup white beans, soaked
- ⅓ cup frozen green peas
- ½ tablespoon olive oil
- ½ cup frozen chopped green beans
- 1 medium chopped onion
- ½ teaspoon rosemary
- 2 cloves crushed garlic
- ½ teaspoon thyme
- 2 stalks chopped celery
- ½ teaspoon oregano
- 3 medium diced carrots
- ½ teaspoon marjoram
- 1 diced green bell pepper
- ½ cup cooked pasta shells
- 8 cups water
- 1 teaspoon salt
- ½ teaspoon black pepper

Rinse the beans and boil for 20 minutes. Heat the oil in a non-stick skillet and sauté the onion and garlic for 3-4 minutes. Add the celery, carrots and green pepper and continue to cook for 1-2 minutes. Add the water, salt and pepper and bring to boil, cover and simmer for 15 minutes. Add the pasta shells, green beans and peas and continue to cook for 10 minutes. Serve hot.

Notes: Excellent source of Vitamin C, A, B1, Folate and Iron. Good source of Vitamin B6, Calcium and Zinc.

Serving Size: 6
Prep Time: 1:00

Calories 192	Carbohydrate 35g	Cholesterol 0mg
Protein 11g	Fat 1g	Dietary Fiber 8g
	% Calories from fat 7%	

SOUPS

Miso Soup

    2 ounces inaka miso (country style)
    3 cups dashi stock**
    5 ounces silken bean curd diced

Put dashi stock into a pan. Add miso and stir until dissolved. Add bean curd and heat. Do not allow to boil. Serve garnished with finely sliced green onions.

    **Dashi Stock
    50 grams dried bonito flakes
    2.5 x 1.5 inches dried kelp
    7 cups water

Wipe the kelp with a damp cloth. Cover with water and heat. Just before the water boils remove the kelp and discard. Sprinkle bonito flakes and strain as the flakes begin to sink.

Note: Good source of Vitamin B12

Serving Size: 4
Prep Time: 0:15

Calories 58	Carbohydrates 5g	Cholesterol 3mg
Protein 6g	Fat 2g	Dietary Fiber 1g
	% Calories from fat 31%	

SOUPS

Phytomineral Soup

- 1 medium chopped onion
- ½ cup firm tofu
- 2 sticks chopped celery
- 2 cups spinach leaves, chopped
- 4 cloves crushed garlic
- ½ cup chopped parsley
- 1 teaspoon curry powder
- 1 teaspoon thyme
- 2 medium sliced carrots
- ½ teaspoon rosemary
- ½ cup corn
- 1 tablespoon olive oil
- 1 15 ounce can of tomatoes
- 5 cups water
- 1 packet vegetable bouillon cube
- Pinch salt
- 1 cup frozen peas
- ¼ teaspoon black pepper

Heat the oil in a large non-stick skillet. Sauté the onions and garlic for 3-5 minutes. Add the celery and carrots and sauté for a further 2 minutes. Add the corn, tomatoes, parsley, thyme, rosemary and sage. Dissolve the packet of vegetable broth in a cup of boiling water. Add to the pan with 4 more cups of water. Bring to a boil, cover and reduce the heat. Simmer for 20 minutes. Add the peas, tofu and spinach. Season to taste and simmer for 5 more minutes.

Notes: Excellent source of Vitamin C, A, B6, Folate and Iron. Good source of Vitamin B1, B2, Niacin, Calcium and Zinc.

Serving Size: 6
Prep Time: 0:30

Calories 153	Carbohydrate 23g	Cholesterol 0mg
Protein 7g	Fat 4g	Dietary Fiber 4g
	% Calories from fat 24%	

SOUPS

Rice and Celery Soup

- 6 sticks celery, finely chopped
- 1 15 ounce can of tomatoes
- 1 cup rice
- 1 tablespoon extra virgin olive oil
- 2 chicken bouillon cubes
- ½ teaspoon salt
- 6 cups water
- ⅓ cup fresh parsley, finely chopped
- ½ medium chopped onion
- ½ teaspoon black pepper

Crumble and dissolve the chicken bouillon cubes in water and heat in a saucepan. In a skillet, heat the oil and sauté the onion and garlic for 3-4 minutes. Add the celery, finely chopped tomatoes, salt and pepper. Cook on low heat, stirring frequently for 10-15 minutes. Add the rice and continue heating for 20 minutes or until the rice is cooked. Remove from heat, add the fresh parsley and serve.

Notes: Excellent source of Vitamin C. Good source of Vitamin A, B6, B1, Folate, Niacin and Iron.

Serving Size: 6
Prep Time: 0:40

Calories 158	Carbohydrate 30g	Cholesterol 0mg
Protein 4g	Fat 2g	Dietary Fiber 2g
	% Calories from fat 15%	

SOUPS

Root Vegetable Soup

- 2 carrots, peeled and diced
- 1 tablespoon parsley
- 1 turnip, peeled and diced
- 1 teaspoon olive oil
- 1 rutabaga, peeled and diced
- 3 cups water
- 1 parsnip, peeled and diced
- ¼ teaspoon sea salt
- 1 onion, chopped
- ¼ teaspoon black pepper
- 2 cloves garlic, crushed

Heat a large non-stick skillet and sauté the onion and garlic in olive oil. Add the turnip and parsnip and continue to sauté for 5 minutes. Add the carrot and sauté for 3 minutes. Add the water and bring to a boil. Cover and simmer for 30 minutes or until cooked. Adjust the seasonings and serve hot, garnished with fresh parsley.

Notes: Excellent source of Vitamin C, A and Folate. Good source of Vitamin B6 and B1. 1/2 cup of nonfat sour cream may be added to the cooked soup to increase the calcium content of the soup.

Serving Size: 4
Prep Time: 0:40

Calories 82	Carbohydrate 17g	Cholesterol 0mg
Protein 2g	Fat 1g	Dietary Fiber 5g
	% Calories from fat 14%	

Tomato Soup

- 12 medium tomatoes
- ½ teaspoon pepper
- 1 large onion, chopped
- ½ teaspoon Tabasco sauce
- 3 tablespoons tomato paste
- ½ teaspoon salt
- 3 cups chicken broth
- 1 teaspoon fresh basil
- 1 teaspoon sugar

Combine the finely chopped and peeled tomatoes, onion, chicken broth and tomato paste in a large saucepan. Bring to a boil, reduce the heat, cover and simmer for 15-20 minutes. Cool and blend until smooth. Return to the pan, add the seasonings and heat through. Serve garnished with finely chopped fresh tomato.

Notes: Excellent source of Vitamin C, A, Folate and Niacin. Good source of Vitamin B6, B1, B2 and Iron.

Serving Size: 6
Prep Time: 0:30

Calories 105	Carbohydrate 16g	Cholesterol 1mg
Protein 8g	Fat 2g	Dietary Fiber 3g
	% Calories from Fat 17%	

BEANS, PASTA AND RICE

Adzuki Beans and Rice

- 1 cup adzuki beans
- 1 tablespoon olive oil
- 1 medium onion
- 1 cup rice
- 2 cloves garlic
- ½ cup vegetable broth
- 1 teaspoon salt
- ¼ teaspoon chili powder

Wash beans and cover with water. Bring to a boil, remove from heat and let soak for one hour. Drain and add sufficient cold water to cover the beans. Add chopped onion, crushed garlic cloves and salt. Canned beans may be used. Bring to the boil and simmer for 1½ hours until tender. Add extra water if necessary. Place bean mixture in a blender and purée till smooth. Cook rice using broth as the liquid. Add chili powder to cooked rice and set aside. Heat olive oil in a heavy skillet and add puréed bean mixture. Simmer for 5 minutes, stirring frequently. Stir in rice and heat for a further 5 minutes. Serve with a fresh salad.

Notes: Excellent source of Vitamin B1, Folate, Niacin, Iron and Zinc. Good source of Vitamin A and B6.

Serves: 4
Prep Time: 2:00 hours (0:20)

Calories 390	Carbohydrate 73g	Cholesterol 0mg
Protein 14g	Fat 4g	Dietary Fiber 8g
	% Calories from fat 10%	

Baked Beans

    3 cups pinto beans, canned
    ½ teaspoon mustard powder
    1 large onion
    1 teaspoon chili powder
    1 15 ounce can of tomato sauce
    1 teaspoon honey

Preheat oven to 350°F. Chop onion and add to beans, tomatoes, onions, honey and seasonings. Bake in an oiled, uncovered casserole dish for an hour. This may be kept warm in a covered pot. Serve with hot bread and a mixed salad.

Optional: Add one cup chopped apple (with peel on).

Notes: Excellent source of Folate. Good source of Vitamin C, A, B6, B1, B2, Iron and Zinc.

    Serves: 4
    Prep Time: 1:00

Calories 174	Carbohydrate 34g	Cholesterol 0mg
Protein 10	Fat 2g	Dietary Fiber 8g
	% Calories from fat 4%	

Bean, Noodle and Nut Casserole

- 12 ounces noodles
- 4 medium onions
- 1 pound blackeyed peas
- 4 ounces cashews
- ½ tablespoon olive oil
- 4 ounces peanuts

Wash blackeyed peas. Boil 4 cups of water and drop the blackeyed peas in. Boil for 2 minutes. Set aside to soak for one hour. Cook noodles according to package instructions. Sauté onions in olive oil until clear and soft. Toss nuts with onions in the frying pan until browned lightly. Drain blackeyed peas and cover with 4 cups of cold water. Bring back to a boil and simmer for 30 minutes or until tender. Combine drained noodles, blackeyed peas, onions and nuts in a casserole dish. Cover and heat for 20 minutes in a 350º oven. Serve with tomato sauce and a fresh salad.

Notes: Excellent source of Vitamin B6, B12, B1, B2, Folate, Niacin, Iron and Zinc. Good source of Calcium. This is a satisfying vegetarian entree.

Serves: 10
Prep Time: 2:30 (20 minutes)
Reduce the prep time by 2 hours using canned beans.

Calories 429	Carbohydrate 59g	Cholesterol 0mg
Protein 21g	Fat 14g	Dietary Fiber 8g
	% Calories from Fat 28%	

BEANS, PASTA AND RICE

Blackeyed Peas

    2 quarts water
    1 pound ground turkey
    1 pound blackeyed peas
    2 cloves garlic, crushed
    1 medium onion
    1 teaspoon garlic powder
    1 teaspoon salt
    1 pinch baking soda
    1 red pepper pod, crushed

Bring water to boil. Add washed blackeyed peas, onion, garlic, salt, garlic powder and crushed red pepper pod. Cook on low heat until the peas are tender (about one hour). Mash the peas with a large wooden spoon then add ground turkey, ginger and baking soda. Adjust water to give a mushy consistency.

Notes: Excellent source of Vitamin B6, B1, Folate, Niacin, Iron and Zinc. Good source of Vitamin C, B2 and Calcium.

Serves: 6
Prep Time: 1:30 (15 minutes)
Reduce the prep time by 1 hour by using canned peas

Calories 376	Carbohydrate 48g	Cholesterol 60mg
Protein 31g	Fat 7g	Dietary Fiber 8g
	% Calories from fat 17%	

Brown Rice Pilaf

- ¾ cup brown rice
- 1 medium onion, chopped
- 2 cups vegetable broth
- 3 cloves garlic, crushed
- 1 package frozen peas
- 1 tablespoon olive oil
- 1 chopped red bell pepper

Heat the oil in a non-stick skillet. Sauté onions and garlic for 3-5 minutes. Add the brown rice and vegetable broth. Bring to a boil and boil for 5 minutes. Turn down the heat, cover the pan and simmer for 40 minutes. Check the level of liquid occasionally and add extra if necessary. Boil the peas and chopped peppers for 3 minutes and add the rice mixture. Mix thoroughly. Goes well with chicken or a bean dish.

Notes: Excellent source of Vitamin C, A, B6, B1, Folate and Iron. Good source of Vitamin B2, Niacin and Zinc.

Optional extra for added protein: Add 1 cup diced chicken.

Serving Size: 6
Prep Time: 1:15

Calories 188	Carbohydrate 33g	Cholesterol 1mg
Protein 5g	Fat 4g	Dietary Fiber 2g
	% Calories from fat 20%	

Flageolets (Small French Green Beans)

- 2 cups flageolets, soaked
- 2 cloves garlic, crushed
- 4 cups water
- ½ teaspoon salt
- 1 tablespoon olive oil
- ½ teaspoon black pepper
- 1 medium onion, chopped
- 1 tablespoon parsley, chopped

Soak flageolets overnight. Drain and rinse. Heat the water in a pot. Heat the olive oil in a large skillet. Sauté the onion and garlic until lightly browned and soft (about 5 minutes). Stir in the drained flageolets and heat for 3 minutes over a low flame. Add the hot water and cover the pan. Simmer for one hour. Add extra water if necessary. Adjust seasoning and serve sprinkled with fresh, chopped parsley.

Notes: Excellent source of Vitamin B1, Folate, Iron and Zinc. Good source of Vitamin B6 and Calcium.

Serves: 6
Prep Time: 1:30
Reduce prep time to 10 minutes by using canned beans.

Calories 228	Carbohydrate 42g	Cholesterol 0mg
Protein 13g	Fat 3g	Dietary Fiber 12g
	% Calories from fat 10%	

BEANS, PASTA AND RICE

Lemon Rice

- 1 ½ cups long-grain rice
- 1 tablespoon fresh parsley
- 1 ½ cups water
- 1 medium onion, chopped fine
- 2 tablespoons fresh lemon juice
- ¼ teaspoon fresh dill
- 1 tablespoon olive oil

Heat a non-stick skillet and spray with olive oil. Sauté the onion for 2-3 minutes until transparent. Add the rice and dill. Cover with the water. Simmer covered for 20-30 minutes until cooked. Add the fresh lemon juice and season to taste. Serve garnished with parsley.

Serving Size: 4
Prep Time: 0:30

Calories 224	Carbohydrate 48g	Cholesterol 0mg
Protein 1g	Fat 3g	Dietary Fiber <1g
	% Calories from fat 14%	

Lentil and Pecan Casserole

- 2 cups lentils
- ½ cup pecans
- 1 tablespoon olive oil
- 1 teaspoon soy sauce
- ¼ teaspoon thyme
- 1 tablespoon cheddar cheese, shredded

Soak beans overnight in cold water. Drain and bring to the boil. Simmer until tender. Preheat the oven to 350°F. Crush the beans. Add chopped pecans and seasonings. Place in an oiled skillet. Heat for 15 minutes. Add grated cheese and continue until melted (3-5 minutes). Serve with a green salad.

Notes: Excellent source of Vitamin B6, B1, Folate, Iron and Zinc. Good source of Vitamin C, B2 and Niacin.

Serves: 4
Prep Time: 2:00
Reduce prep time to 10 minutes by using canned lentils.

Calories 435	Carbohydrate 58g	Cholesterol 0mg
Protein 29g	Fat 12g	Dietary Fiber 30g
	% Calories from fat 24%	

BEANS, PASTA AND RICE

Lentil Patties

- 1 cup lentils, canned
- ¼ teaspoon ground cumin
- 1 medium onion
- ½ teaspoon curry powder
- 1 tablespoon olive oil
- 1 pinch celery salt
- 1 clove garlic
- ¾ cup bread crumbs
- ½ teaspoon salt
- 1 tablespoon liquid egg substitute or 1 egg

Preheat oven to 350°F. Stir lentils and seasonings together in a bowl. Add half of the bread crumbs. Lightly beat the egg with a fork and add to the mixture to bind (this step is optional). Using wet hands mold the lentil mixture into 8 evenly shaped patties. Place the remaining bread crumbs into a large plastic bag. Add the patties and roll them in the crumbs inside the bag until evenly covered. Remove the patties and set aside. Heat the olive oil in a skillet and lightly fry the patties to brown them. Place the skillet in the oven and bake for 20 minutes. Serve with a tomato or yogurt based sauce.

Notes: Excellent source of Vitamin B6, B1, Folate and Iron. Good source of Vitamin B2, Niacin and Zinc.

Serves: 4
Prep Time: 0:30

Calories 303	Carbohydrate 44g	Cholesterol 53mg
Protein 18g	Fat 3g	Dietary Fiber 16g
	% Calories from fat 9%	

Mexican Bean Pie

- 4 corn tortillas
- 2 tomatoes, chopped
- ½ cup scallions, sliced thin
- 2 teaspoons chili powder
- 2 cloves garlic, crushed
- 1 teaspoon coriander ground
- 2 green bell peppers, diced
- ½ cup egg substitute, liquid
- 1 tablespoon olive oil
- ¼ cup cheddar cheese, shredded
- 2 cups pinto beans, cooked, mashed

Heat tortillas for 5-8 minutes over a flame or in a hot oven. Place in a blender or pestle and mortar and crumble finely. Take 4 pie pans (5" in diameter) and spray or coat with olive oil. Coat with the tortilla crumbs, setting aside extra for topping. Heat the rest of the olive oil in a heavy skillet and sauté the scallions, peppers and garlic for about 3-4 minutes, until tender. Add the beans, tomatoes, chili powder and coriander and continue to sauté for a further 5 minutes. Remove from the heat and stir in the egg substitute. Divide among the prepared pans and sprinkle the tops with the rest of the crumbs. Bake at 375°F for 20 minutes. Top with cheese and melt for a further few minutes in the hot oven. Serve with a salad.

Notes: Excellent source of Vitamin C, A, B6, B1, Folate and Iron. Good source of Vitamin B2, Calcium and Zinc.

Serves: 4
Prep Time: 0:45

Calories 281	Carbohydrate 41g	Cholesterol 2mg
Protein 15g	Fat 6g	Dietary Fiber 11g
	% Calories from fat 21%	

BEANS, PASTA AND RICE

Navy Bean Stew

- ½ pound navy beans
- 1 stalk celery
- 2 tablespoons olive oil
- ¼ teaspoon black pepper
- 1 large onion
- ¼ cup parsley sprigs
- 1 clove garlic
- 1 teaspoon dried basil
- ½ cup tomato sauce
- 4 cups water
- 1 medium carrot

Soak rinsed and sorted navy beans in water overnight or use the short method by covering with 2 ½ cups of cold water, bringing to a boil for 2 minutes and then letting stand for one hour. Drain. Canned beans may be used. Heat olive oil in large soup pot and sauté chopped onions and crushed garlic clove until lightly browned and moist. Add tomato sauce, thinly sliced carrot, chopped celery, black pepper and simmer for 10 more minutes. Add navy beans and 4 cups of boiling water. Lower the heat and simmer in the covered pot until the beans are tender (about 45 minutes). Serve with hot bread or pasta salad for a nourishing main dish.

Notes: Excellent source of Vitamin C, A, B6, B2, B1, Folate and Iron. Good source of Vitamin B2, Niacin, Calcium and Zinc.

Serves: 4
Prep Time: 0:15 (30)

Calories 279	Carbohydrate 41g	Cholesterol 0mg
Protein 14g	Fat 8g	Dietary Fiber 16g
	% Calories from fat 24%	

Noodles with Tuna

    1 6 ounce can tuna in water
    ¼ teaspoon salt
    1   tablespoon fresh lemon juice
    ¼ teaspoon black pepper
    ¾ pound linguini
    1 tablespoon virgin olive oil
    4   quarts water

Cook the pasta for 8-9 minutes until tender. Drain well and lay in a warm serving dish. While the pasta is cooking, prepare the tuna sauce. Drain the tuna and mix with the lemon juice and olive oil. Season to taste and set on top of the linguini. Sprinkle a little grated Parmesan or Romano cheese on the top.

Notes: Excellent source of Vitamin B12, B1 and Niacin. Good source of Vitamin B2 and Iron.

    Serving Size: 4
    Prep Time: 0:45

Calories 321	Carbohydrate 45g	Cholesterol 63mg
Protein 21g	Fat 6g	Dietary Fiber 2g
	% Calories from fat 16%	

BEANS, PASTA AND RICE

Pasta and Eggplant

- 2 tablespoons olive oil
- ¼ teaspoon hot chili peppers
- ½ lb fresh pasta
- ½ teaspoon salt
- 1 eggplant, peeled and chopped
- ½ teaspoon black pepper
- ½ onion
- 4 cloves crushed garlic
- 2 tablespoons fresh parsley
- 1 28 ounces can of tomatoes
- 1 tablespoon grated Parmesan

Cook the pasta by boiling in salted water until tender. Meanwhile, heat one tablespoon of the oil in a large non-stick skillet and sauté the onion and garlic for 3-5 minutes. Add half of the eggplant and cook for 8-10 minutes until tender. Remove and keep warm. Heat the rest of the olive oil and cook the remainder of the eggplant. Add the tomatoes, chili peppers and seasoning. Return the eggplant to the pan and warm the whole mixture. Drain the pasta and serve with the sauce on top. Garnish with fresh parsley. Serve the Parmesan cheese separately.

Notes: Excellent source of Vitamin C, A, B6, B1, B2, Folate, Niacin and Iron. Good source of Calcium and Zinc.

Serving Size: 1
Prep Time: 0:30

Calories 434	Carbohydrate 79g	Cholesterol 84mg
Protein 17g	Fat 7g	Dietary Fiber 5g
	% Calories from fat 14%	

Pasta Primavera

- 1 pound pea pods or mange tout
- ½ cup diced red bell pepper
- 1 pound asparagus
- ½ cup diced yellow pepper
- 1 cup green beans, sliced
- 2 tablespoons chopped chives
- ½ cup carrots sliced thin
- 4 tablespoons chopped parsley
- 1 tablespoon olive oil
- ¾ pound angel hair pasta

Bring a large pot of salted water to the boil. Blanch the pea pods, asparagus, green beans and carrots separately by dipping for 30 seconds and placing in ice cold water immediately afterwards for 30 seconds. Drain and pat dry. Save the cooking water. Heat the olive oil in a large skillet and sauté the bell peppers. Add the blanched vegetables and continue to heat for another 1-2 minutes. Re-boil the water and cook the pasta for 3-4 minutes, drain and transfer to a warm serving bowl. Add the hot vegetables and chives, toss and season to taste. Serve the pasta on individual pasta dishes and pass fresh grated Parmesan cheese for topping.

Notes: Excellent source of Vitamin C, A, B6, B1, B2, Folate, Niacin and Iron. Good source of Zinc.

Serving Size: 6
Prep Time: 0:40

Calories 296	Carbohydrate 55g	Cholesterol 0mg
Protein 12g	Fat 3g	Dietary Fiber 6g
	% Calories from fat 9%	

BEANS, PASTA AND RICE

Quinoa-Nut Vegetable Pilaf

- 1 cup quinoa, rinsed and drained
- 1 medium diced carrot
- 1 tablespoon olive oil
- 2 tablespoons almonds, toasted and chopped
- 1 medium chopped onion
- 1 clove crushed garlic
- 2 tablespoons chopped parsley

Rinse the quinoa under cold running water for 4-5 minutes to remove the grit and bitter flavorings. Heat the olive oil in a large, non-stick pan and sauté the onion and garlic for 3-5 minutes until transparent. Add the carrot and continue to cook in the covered pan for 2-3 minutes more. Add the quinoa, water and salt and boil for 2 minutes. Reduce the heat, cover the pot and simmer for 20 minutes until tender. Add the chopped, toasted almonds and mix well. Add additional water if necessary so that the pilaf is moist. Serve hot.

Notes: Excellent source of Vitamin A and Iron. Good source of Vitamin B6, B1, B2, Folate and Zinc.

Serving Size: 4
Prep Time: 1:00

Calories 218	Carbohydrate 34g	Cholesterol 0mg
Protein 7g	Fat 6g	Dietary Fiber 4g
	% Calories from fat 25%	

Risotto

    1 cup rice
    ½ tablespoon extra virgin olive oil
    1¾ cups vegetable broth
    1 teaspoon white wine
    ½ medium chopped onion

Heat the oil in a non-stick pan and sauté the onion and garlic for 3-4 minutes until transparent. Add the rice and vegetable broth and bring to a boil. Boil for a minute, then reduce the heat, cover the pan and simmer for 25 minutes or until tender. Add extra water if necessary. Serve hot.

Notes: Excellent source of Vitamin A and B12. Good source of Niacin, Iron and Zinc. Optional Extras: ½ teaspoon of powdered saffron or ½ cup of Porcini mushrooms (sliced and sautéed with the onions and garlic).

Serving Size: 4
Prep Time: 0:40

Calories 260	Carbohydrate 49g	Cholesterol 1mg
Protein 6g	Fat 4g	Dietary Fiber 2g
	% Calories from fat 13%	

BEANS, PASTA AND RICE

Spaghetti with Artichoke Hearts

- 1 14 ounce can of artichoke hearts
- ½ teaspoon salt
- 2 cloves crushed garlic
- ½ teaspoon black pepper, fresh ground
- 1 small chopped onion
- ¼ cup grated Parmesan cheese
- 2 tablespoons olive oil
- 2 egg whites
- 3 tablespoons fresh chopped parsley
- ¼ pound spaghetti
- ½ teaspoon basil

Rinse and quarter the canned artichoke hearts. Heat the olive oil in a skillet and sauté the onion and garlic for 3-4 minutes. Add ½ cup water, parsley, basil, salt and pepper. Simmer for 15 minutes. Boil a large pot of salted water and cook the spaghetti for 8-10 minutes or until cooked. Combine the egg whites and parmesan cheese. Toss the pasta in the mixture. Add the artichoke mixture and reheat. Add extra water if it is too dry. Serve with extra Parmesan cheese as a topping.

Notes: Excellent source of Vitamin C, B12, B2, Folate, Niacin and Iron. Good source of Vitamin B6, Calcium and Zinc.

Serving Size: 4
Prep Time: 0:30

Calories 355	Carbohydrate 56g	Cholesterol 4mg
Protein 14g	Fat 9g	Dietary Fiber 7g
	% Calories from fat 23%	

Southern Style Beans and Rice

- 1 cup canned red kidney beans
- ¼ teaspoon black pepper
- 1 medium onion, chopped
- 1 clove garlic
- ½ teaspoon Cajun seasoning
- 1 small green bell pepper
- 1 cup rice
- 1 pinch salt

Drain and rinse the beans. Meanwhile cook the rice by covering with ½ inch of water and simmer in a covered pan until the water has been absorbed and the rice is cooked. Sauté the onion, garlic and chopped pepper for 6-8 minutes until browned and cooked. Add the beans and sufficient water to make a thick gravy. Season with the Cajun seasoning, salt and freshly ground black pepper. Serve with the rice.

Notes: Excellent source of Vitamin C, B1 and Folate. Good source of Vitamin B6, Niacin, Iron and Zinc.

Serves: 6
Prep Time: 0:20

Calories 224	Carbohydrate 46g	Cholesterol 0mg
Protein 10g	Fat 1g	Dietary Fiber 6g
	% Calories from fat 2%	

BEANS, PASTA AND RICE

Stir-fry Vegetables and Rice

- 1 medium chopped onion
- ½ teaspoon black pepper
- 1 peeled and chopped carrot
- ½ red bell pepper
- 1 cup Mung bean sprouts
- 2 sliced water chestnuts
- 1 cup bok choy, sliced thick
- 1 teaspoon sesame oil
- ¼ cup slivered almonds
- 2 cups cooked brown rice
- 2 tablespoons soy sauce

Heat the sesame oil in a large wok or deep skillet. Add the chopped onion and carrot and stir-fry for 2 minutes. Add the other vegetables and continue to stir-fry for 3-4 minutes more. Add the almonds, soy sauce and pepper. Serve with the cooked rice.

Notes: Excellent source of Vitamin C, A, B6 and Folate. Good source of Vitamin B1, Niacin and Zinc.

Serving Size: 4
Prep Time: 0:10

Calories 210	Carbohydrate 33g	Cholesterol 0mg
Protein 6g	Fat 7g	Dietary Fiber 3g
	% Calories from fat 28%	

Tasty Rice and Tofu

    1 ½   pounds tofu, low-fat
    1   teaspoon fresh basil
    ½ tablespoon olive oil
    ½ teaspoon thyme
    2 cloves crushed garlic
    ¼ teaspoon marjoram
    2 medium chopped onions
    ¼ teaspoon savory
    1 cup sliced mushrooms
    2 cups vegetable broth
    ⅓ cup Tamari soy sauce
    2 cups cooked rice
    A dash Tabasco sauce

Heat the olive oil in a nonstick skillet. Add the garlic and onions and sauté for 3-5 minutes until transparent. Add the mushrooms and cook 2 more minutes, shaking the skillet constantly. Remove the vegetables and set aside on a warm dish. Cut the tofu into 1 ½ inch size cubes. In a mixing bowl combine the Tamari, basil, thyme, savory, marjoram and Tabasco. Dip the tofu cubes in the mixture and brown the cubes in the skillet. Add the vegetable broth to the skillet and return the vegetable mixture. Simmer for 10 minutes and serve hot with rice as a main dish.

Notes: Excellent source of Vitamin A and Iron. Good source of Vitamin B6, B1, B2, Folate, Niacin, Calcium and Zinc.

    Serving Size: 6
    Prep Time: 0:20

FISH

Baked Red Snapper

    4   pounds red snapper
    1   teaspoon sugar
    ½   tablespoon olive oil
    1   tablespoon Worcestershire sauce
    ½   tablespoon butter
    ¼   cup white wine
    1   medium chopped onion
    8   fluid ounces tomato sauce
    3   sticks chopped celery
    ½   teaspoon Creole seasoning
    1   medium green bell pepper
       pinch of salt
    4   cloves crushed garlic
       pinch black pepper, fresh ground

Season the fish and place in an ovenproof dish. Melt the olive oil and butter and sauté the onions, celery, green bell pepper and garlic for 5-8 minutes. Add the tomato sauce, Worcestershire sauce and season to taste. Cook slowly for one hour. Heat the oven to 300°F. Pour the wine over the fish and then the sauce. Place in the oven with a small piece of aluminum foil loosely on top. Cook for one hour, basting occasionally. Serve with rice or mashed potatoes as a main dish.

Notes: Excellent source of Vitamin C, B12. Good source of Vitamin B6.

Serving Size: 8
Prep Time: 0:20
Baking Time: 2:00

Calories 85	Carbohydrate 6g	Cholesterol 18mg
Protein 10g	Fat 2g	Dietary Fiber 1g
	% Calories from fat 24%	

Baked Salmon

- 1   4 pound salmon
- 4   black peppercorns
- 1   medium sliced carrot
- 1   sprig parsley
- 1   medium sliced onion
- 1   bay leaf
- 1   Tablespoon butter

Place the salmon on a large piece of aluminum foil in an ovenproof dish. Slice the carrot and onion and arrange on top of the fish with the peppercorns, parsley and bay leaf. Dab with butter and wrap the foil around the fish. Add the water to the base of the dish and place in a cool oven (250°F) and cook for 2 to 3 hours until cooked through but not dry. Serve hot with Hollandaise Sauce, garnished with lemon wedges. Serve cold, garnished with thinly sliced cucumber, lemon slices and parsley. Cold salmon goes well with mayonnaise or a yogurt dressing.

Notes: Excellent source of Vitamin C, A, B6, B12, Calcium and Iron. Good source of Niacin.

Serving Size: 4
Prep Time: 0:15
Baking Time: 2:00

Calories 493	Carbohydrate 2g	Cholesterol 18mg
Protein 47g	Fat 32g	Dietary Fiber 0.5g
	% Calories from fat 58%	

FISH

Barbecued Fish with Tarragon Sauce

    2 medium red snapper
    ½ tablespoon olive oil
    1 tablespoon fennel
    1 tablespoon butter
    1 tablespoon sage
    4 tablespoons white wine
    2 bay leaves
pinch salt
    1 tablespoon rosemary
pinch black pepper
Tarragon Sauce
    4 tablespoons tarragon
    1   cup lemon juice
    ¼ cup butter substitute

Mix the finely chopped herbs except the tarragon together with the butter and place inside each fish. Brush the fish with oil and place in a wire fish barbecue griller. Grill over hot coals. Combine the ingredients for the tarragon sauce and warm in a small pan. Serve hot as a main dish.

Notes: Excellent source of Vitamin C and B12. Good source of Vitamin A, B6, Calcium and Iron.

Serving Size: 4
Prep Time: 0:20

Calories 148	Carbohydrate 9.g	Cholesterol 28mg
Protein 10g	Fat 6g	Dietary Fiber <1g
	% Calories from fat 40%	

Broiled Orange Roughy

- 2 orange roughy fillets
- 1 teaspoon sugar
- 6 medium tomatoes
- ¼ cup red wine vinegar
- 1 medium red onion
- ½ tablespoon olive oil
- 2 cucumbers, peeled
- ½ teaspoon ground pepper
- 1 teaspoon salt
- 2 medium carrots, diced
- 2 tablespoons tarragon
- ¼ cup frozen green peas

Remove the core and seeds from the tomatoes and chop coarsely. Combine with the onion, cucumber, finely chopped tarragon, salt, sugar and chill. Season the orange roughy fillets with salt and fresh ground black pepper and brush (or spray) with olive oil. Broil for 2-3 minutes until cooked. At the same time place the diced carrots in a small saucepan and cover with cold water. Bring to the boil and simmer for 2 minutes. Add the frozen peas and continue to cook for another 2-3 minutes. Drain and set aside. Place the fish on a warm serving dish. Combine the peas and carrots with ½ cup of the chilled relish and arrange the vegetable mixture around the fish. Serve the rest of the relish as a side dish. Serve the fish hot with garlic mashed potatoes.

Notes: Excellent source of Vitamin A, C, B6, B1, B2, Folate and Iron.

Serving Size: 2
Prep Time: 0:20

Calories 205	Carbohydrate 39g	Cholesterol 10mg
Protein 7g	Fat 5g	Dietary Fiber 9g
	% Calories from Fat 20%	

Sole

- 1 pound Dover sole fillets
- 2 tablespoons Dijon mustard
- 1 small onion, chopped fine
- 2 tablespoons olive oil
- 4 tablespoons nonfat yogurt
- 1 teaspoon fresh chopped tarragon

Preheat the oven to 425°F. Spray a shallow non-stick ovenproof dish with olive oil spray and arrange the onion slices in the pan. Place the fish over the onion slices. Combine the yogurt, mustard, olive oil and tarragon and season to taste with salt and pepper. Spread over the fish. Bake uncovered for 7-9 minutes. Serve hot with brown rice or small potatoes.

Notes: Good source of Niacin and Calcium. This dish is relatively high in fat because there is virtually no carbohydrate in white fish. It is a nutritious supper dish, low in calories and delicious.

Serving Size: 4
Prep Time: 0:15

Calories 158	Carbohydrate 3g	Cholesterol 0mg
Protein 19g	Fat 8g	Dietary Fiber 2g
	% Calories from fat 44%	

FISH

Ginger-Sesame Salmon

 4 salmon steaks
 1 tablespoon fresh ginger root
 1 teaspoon fresh lemon juice
 2 green onions, cut in strips
 1 cup water
 1 clove garlic, crushed
 2 teaspoons soy sauce
 1 tablespoon sesame oil
 2 teaspoons rice vinegar

Place the water and fresh lemon juice in a deep non-stick sauté pan or skillet. Bring to a boil. Place the salmon steaks in the water and cover the pan. Reduce the heat and simmer very gently for 6-8 minutes until the fish is opaque in color. Arrange the salmon on a warm serving dish. Mix the soy sauce, rice vinegar and finely grated ginger together and spoon over the salmon. Cut the green onions into thin strips and scatter over the top of the fish. In a small pan combine the garlic and sesame oil. Warm the mixture until it browns and drizzle over the top of the fish. Serve hot.

Notes: Excellent source of Vitamin C, B6, B12, B1, Folate and Niacin. Good source of Vitamin B2, Iron and Zinc.

 Serving Size: 4
 Prep Time: 0:20

Calories 254	Carbohydrate 6g	Cholesterol 88mg
Protein 36g	Fat 9g	Dietary Fiber 2g
	% Calories from fat 33%	

FISH

Grilled Tuna

    4   medium tuna steaks
    ½ tablespoon olive oil
    pinch of salt
    ¼ teaspoon black pepper

Brush the tuna steaks with olive oil and season with salt and pepper. Place a rack 4" from the broiler and heat for 10 minutes. Broil the steaks 4 minutes on each side. Serve on a bed of brown rice with warm cilantro sauce.

Notes: Excellent source of Vitamin A, B6, B12, B1, B2 and Niacin.

Serving Size: 4
Prep Time: 0:20

Calories 260	Carbohydrate 1g	Cholesterol 65mg
Protein 40g	Fat 10g	Dietary Fiber 0g
	% Calories from fat 36%	

Halibut with Broccoli and Almonds

- ¾ pound halibut fillet
- 2 teaspoons sesame oil
- 2 tablespoons corn starch
- 1 clove garlic
- ½ pound broccoli florets
- ½ teaspoon ginger
- ½ cup julienned carrots
- 2 tablespoons almond slivers
- ¼ cup low-sodium soy sauce
- 2 ½ cups brown rice

Cut halibut into 1 inch by 2 inch strips and coat with corn starch. Combine broccoli, carrots, soy sauce, garlic and ginger in a mixing bowl and set aside. In a large non-stick skillet heat 2 teaspoons of sesame oil, add the fish and fry for 4 to 5 minutes until lightly browned. Remove the fish and set aside. Add the rest of the sesame oil and stir-fry the vegetable mixture for 3 to 4 minutes. Add the almonds and continue to cook for a further minute. Add the fish back to the mixture and warm through for one minute. Serve with the brown rice as a main dish.

Notes: Excellent source of Vitamin C, A, B6, B12, B1, Folate, Niacin, Iron and Zinc. Good source of Vitamin B2 and Calcium.

Serving Size: 4
Prep Time: 0:20

Calories 590
Protein 30g

Carbohydrate 101g
Fat 8g
% Calories from fat 12%

Cholesterol 27mg
Dietary Fiber 3g

FISH

Monkfish, Mushrooms and Lentils

- 2 pounds monkfish
- 2 tablespoons fresh parsley
- 1 tablespoon flour
- 2 cups Porcini mushrooms
- 1 cup lentils
- 1 ½ cups water
- 1 medium onion
- 2 teaspoons corn flour
- 1 bay leaf
- ½ cup white wine
- 1 leek
- 1 tablespoon olive oil
- 2 cloves garlic
- 1 tablespoon butter

Place the lentils and bay leaf in a pan with the water. Bring to a boil, cover and simmer for 20-30 minutes until the lentils are cooked. Set aside, still covered. Melt the oil and butter in a wide skillet. Add chopped onion, leek and garlic and sauté for 5 minutes. Add chopped parsley and continue to cook gently for a further 5 minutes. Add the porcini mushrooms and cook for 4-5 minutes more. Stir in the wine and cook for another minute. Add the filleted monkfish, dipped in seasoned flour. Simmer for 4 minutes on each side. Lift the fish out of the skillet and arrange on a large ovenproof dish. Cover and leave in a warm oven for 10 minutes. Mix 2 teaspoons of corn flour in 2 tablespoons of water and add to the skillet. Stir over a medium heat until the mixture thickens into a coating sauce. Serve the fish on a bed of lentils, covered with the porcini mushroom sauce.

Notes: Excellent source of Vitamin B6, B1, B2, Folate, Niacin, Iron and Zinc. Good source of Vitamin C.

Serving Size: 4
Prep Time: 1:00

Calories 312	Carbohydrate 39g	Cholesterol 18mg
Protein 22g	Fat 8g	Dietary Fiber 7g
	% Calories from fat 22%	

Sea Bass with Apples

    4 medium sea bass steaks
    1 15 ounce can of tomatoes, chopped
    2 medium red apples
    ½ cup vegetable broth
    2 sticks celery, chopped
    ¼ teaspoon salt
    2 medium onions, chopped
    ¼ teaspoon black pepper
    4 teaspoons chopped parsley
    Pinch dill
    1 medium green bell pepper, chopped

Preheat the oven to 350ºF. Place the celery, onions, tomatoes and broth into a pan and cook for 5 minutes. Core and dice the apple and add to the ingredients. Add the parsley and dill and season to taste. Continue cooking a further 2-3 minutes or until completely cooked. Place the mixture in the bottom of an ovenproof dish with the fish steaks on top. Cover with a loose piece of aluminum foil and bake in the oven at 350ºF for 10-15 minutes until the fish is white and cooked. Garnish with parsley and lemon wedges. Serve hot with brown rice or mashed potato as a main dish.

Notes: Excellent source of Vitamin C, A, B6, B1, Folate and Niacin. Good source of Calcium, Iron and Zinc.

    Serving Size: 4
    Prep Time: 0:30

Calories 233	Carbohydrate 24g	Cholesterol 53mg
Protein 27g	Fat 4g	Dietary Fiber 5g
	% Calories from fat 14%	

Sizzling Monkfish Broccoli and Peanuts

¾ pound monkfish (or other firm white fish)
1 clove garlic
2 tablespoons corn flour
1 teaspoon ground ginger
½ pound broccoli florets
1 teaspoon peanut oil
½ cup julienned carrots
1 tablespoon peanuts
¼ cup low-sodium soy sauce
2 ½ cups brown rice
½ teaspoon sesame oil

Combine the fish, cut into 1" X 2" strips with the corn starch and cover evenly. In another bowl, combine the vegetables, sesame oil and seasoning. Heat 2 teaspoons of the peanut oil in a large skillet and add the fish, cooking until lightly browned (4-5 minutes). Remove the fish and set aside. Heat the remaining teaspoon of peanut oil and stir-fry vegetable mixture and peanuts. Cook for 4 minutes. Place the fish in the mixture and cook covered for another minute. Serve over steamed brown rice.

Notes: Excellent source of Vitamin C, A, B6, B12, Folate and Niacin. Good source of Vitamin B1, B2, Iron and Zinc.

Serving Size: 4
Prep Time: 0:20

Calories 314	Carbohydrate 38g	Cholesterol 33mg
Protein 23g	Fat 7g	Dietary Fiber 3g
	% Calories from fat 22%	

Teriyaki Salmon

- 2 pounds salmon
- 1 teaspoon all-purpose flour
- 1 tablespoon brown sugar
- ½ cup white wine
- ¼ cup soy sauce
- 1 teaspoon mustard
- 1 tablespoon olive oil
- 6 slices pineapple

Combine soy sauce, brown sugar, olive oil, flour, wine and mustard in a small pan. Bring to a boil, and then simmer for 3 minutes. Set aside to cool. Wipe fish and pat dry. Preheat the oven to 320°F. Place the fish in the marinade and refrigerate for 15 minutes. Remove the fish from the refrigerator and place on a non-stick oiled pan. Place a slice of pineapple on each fillet. Heat the marinade and brush the fish with hot marinade. Place in the oven for 15 to 20 minutes until white and cooked. Remove and serve garnished with tomatoes for color. Serve with rice as a main dish.

Notes: Excellent source of Vitamin C, B6, B12, B1, B2, Folate, Niacin and Iron.

Serving Size: 6
Prep Time: 0:45

Calories 407	Carbohydrate 14g	Cholesterol 83mg
Protein 32g	Fat 23g	Dietary Fiber 1.3g
	% Calories from fat 33%	

FISH

Trout with Almonds

- 4 trout
- ½ tablespoon olive oil
- ¼ cup almond slivers
- 1 lemon
- ¼ cup flour
- ¼ teaspoon salt
- ½ tablespoon butter
- ¼ teaspoon black pepper

Roll each prepared trout in the seasoned flour. Heat the oil and butter in a large non-stick skillet. Fry the trout 3-4 minutes on each side. Lift from the pan and set aside in a warm place. Add the almonds to the pan, adding extra oil and butter only if absolutely necessary. When browned, lift from the heat and set aside with the fish. Remove the skillet from the heat and add the lemon juice. Mix well and spoon the almonds and juices over the fish. Serve hot as a main dish.

Notes: Excellent source of Vitamin C, B12, B1 and B2. Good source of Iron.

Serving Size: 4
Prep Time: 0:30

Calories 268	Carbohydrate 11g	Cholesterol 65mg
Protein 21g	Fat 12g	Dietary Fiber <1g
	% Calories from fat 47%	

White Fish with Ginger and Lemon

    4 medium halibut steaks
    1 teaspoon peeled chopped ginger root
    2 tablespoons olive oil
    1 tablespoon grated lemon peel
    2 garlic cloves
    1 cup lemon juice
    3 cups frozen green peas
    2 cups cooked brown rice
    2 sliced scallions

Heat one tablespoon of the olive oil in a large nonstick skillet. Sauté the fish steaks until they turn white. Remove the fish and set aside in a warm place. Add the rest of the oil, peas, scallions, ginger and lemon peel. Cook, stirring frequently until the peas are cooked. Return the fish to the pan and heat thoroughly. Serve on a bed of brown rice. Garnish with lemon wedges and parsley. Serve as a main dish.

Notes: Excellent source of Vitamin C, A, B6, B12, B1, Folate, Niacin and Iron. Good source of Vitamin B2, Calcium and Zinc.

Serving Size: 4
Prep Time: 0:20

Calories 460	Carbohydrate 45g	Cholesterol 54mg
Protein 44g	Fat 11g	Dietary Fiber 6g
	% Calories from fat 23%	

POULTRY

Chicken Curry

- 6 chicken breast halves, skinless
- 6 teaspoons curry powder
- 1 ½ cups chicken broth
- 3 teaspoons oregano
- 5 teaspoons Worcestershire sauce
- 1 teaspoon paprika
- 5 crushed bay leaves
- 2 cloves crushed garlic
- ½ teaspoon Tabasco sauce

Preheat the oven to 350°F. Combine all the ingredients except the chicken breasts in a pan and bring to the boil. Place the chicken in an ovenproof dish and cover with the mixture. Cover the dish and bake for 50 minutes or until done.

Notes: Excellent source of Vitamin B6 and Niacin.

Serving Size: 6
Prep Time: 0:10
Baking Time: 0:50

Calories 139	Carbohydrate 4g	Cholesterol 52mg
Protein 24g	Fat 3g	Dietary Fiber 1g
	% Calories from fat 17%	

Chicken in Soy Sauce

    4 skinless chicken legs
    1 clove crushed garlic
    1 cup soy sauce
    3-4 green onions sliced diagonally
    2 tablespoons honey

Combine the soy sauce, honey and garlic. Marinate the chicken legs for at least 2 hours or overnight. Bake in a covered dish for one hour at 350°F. Serve with rice or mashed potatoes. Sprinkle with onions.

Notes: Excellent source of Vitamin B6, B2 and Niacin. Good source of Vitamin B1 and Folate.

    Serving Size: 4
    Prep Time: 1:00
    Marinate Time: 2:00+

Calories 234	Carbohydrate 14g	Cholesterol 113mg
Protein 32g	Fat 5g	Dietary Fiber <1g
	% Calories from fat 21%	

POULTRY

Chicken with Tarragon

- 2 pounds chicken, skinless
- ½ teaspoon salt
- 1 ½ tablespoon butter
- ½ teaspoon black pepper
- ½ tablespoon olive oil
- 1 clove crushed garlic
- 4 sprigs fresh tarragon

Preheat the oven to 325°F. Crush the garlic into the butter and oil and mix together. Smear this mixture over the breasts of the chicken. Place one sprig of tarragon inside each of the pieces and place them in a baking dish. Cover with a piece of aluminum foil leaving the sides open. Place in the oven for 20 minutes, turning twice. Remove the foil and brown for 5 more minutes or until cooked. Serve with a green salad.

Notes: Excellent source of Vitamin B6 and Niacin. Good source of Vitamin B2 and Iron.

Serving Size: 4
Prep Time: 0:30

Calories 166	Carbohydrate 2g	Cholesterol 70mg
Protein 27g	Fat 5g	Dietary Fiber <1g
	% Calories from fat 28%	

Lemon Chicken and English Walnuts

    4 chicken breast halves, skinless
    2 tablespoons soy sauce
    2 tablespoons fresh lemon juice
    1 tablespoon corn flour
    2 tablespoons chopped walnuts
    ¼ teaspoon white pepper

Preheat the oven to 325°F. Dissolve the corn flour in the soy sauce and lemon juice. Add the white pepper and chopped walnuts. Heat a non-stick skillet sprayed with olive oil and add the chicken breast halves. Brown for 2-3 minutes on each side. Remove and set aside on a warm serving dish. Add the sauce and allow the corn flour to thicken. Adjust the consistency if desired. Pour over the chicken and place in oven for 20 minutes. Serve hot.

Notes: Excellent source of Vitamin B6 and Niacin. Good source of Vitamin B1 and Zinc.

    Serving Size: 4
    Prep Time: 0:10
    Baking Time: 0:20

Calories 166	Carbohydrate 5g	Cholesterol 65mg
Protein 27g	Fat 4g	Dietary Fiber <1g
	% Calories from fat 21%	

POULTRY

Oven-baked Sesame Chicken

- 4 chicken breasts, skinless
- ¼ teaspoon black pepper
- ½ cup flour
- ½ teaspoon paprika
- ¼ cup sesame seeds
- ½ teaspoon salt
- ¼ teaspoon garlic powder
- ¼ cup 1% low-fat milk

Toast sesame seeds in a skillet until golden brown, stirring constantly. Preheat the oven to 400°F. Lightly oil a shallow baking pan. Combine flour, sesame seeds, garlic powder, black pepper, paprika and salt in a bag and shake well. Dip the chicken in milk and then coat in the bag. Place chicken in baking pan and bake for 45 minutes until golden brown.

Notes: Excellent source of Vitamin B6, B1 and Niacin. Good source of Vitamin B2, Folate and Zinc.

Serving Size: 4
Prep Time: 0:10
Baking Time: 0:45

Calories 243	Carbohydrate 14g	Cholesterol 66mg
Protein 31g	Fat 7g	Dietary Fiber <1g
	% Calories from fat 25%	

VEGETABLES AND VEGETARIAN DISHES

Brussels sprouts and Chestnuts

    2 cups Brussels sprouts
    ½ cup roasted chestnuts

Steam Brussels sprouts until just tender (8-10 minutes). Place on a serving dish and arrange warmed roasted chestnuts on top. Serve with roast turkey or chicken.

Notes: Excellent source of Vitamin A, C and Folate. Good source of Vitamin B6.

    Serving Size: 4
    Prep Time: 0:15

Calories 62	Carbohydrate 13g	Cholesterol 0mg
Protein 2g	Fat <1g	Dietary Fiber 4g
	% Calories from fat 7%	

Collard Greens with Pine Nuts

- 1 large bunch collard greens, about 1 ½ pounds
- 1 tablespoon olive oil
- 1 teaspoon butter
- 3 cloves garlic, minced
- 1 tablespoon pine nuts

Rinse collard greens well in a large bowl of cold water. Drain and cut off tough stems. Cut leaves into 1/4-inch strips. Heat olive oil and butter in a heavy deep skillet (avoid overheating). Add the garlic and brown gently. Add pine nuts and continue to cook until lightly toasted. Add the collard greens and cook over a medium heat for a few minutes tossing with a fork. Cover and continue to cook until wilted and tender (about fifteen minutes). Pine nuts (Pignolas) are an excellent source of healthy oils and boost the calorie count of this greens dish. Top with a little soy sauce if desired.

Serving Size: 4
Prep Time: 0:30

Calories 100	Carbohydrate 9g	Cholesterol 2mg
Protein 5g	Fat 6g	Dietary Fiber 6g
	% Calories from fat 54%	

Creamed Spinach

- 2 pounds spinach
- 2 tablespoons water
- 1 teaspoon salt
- ½ cup Greek style plain non fat yogurt
- Fresh ground pepper

Wash the spinach and add the water and salt. Cook in a heavy deep skillet with a lid and shake frequently or lift leaves with a fork. Cook 7-12 minutes until tender and then drain. Add pepper and warmed yogurt and serve hot. A dash of lemon juice or hot sauce may add to the flavor. You may also wish to include mushrooms as these are also full of immune supporting nutrients including beta glucans and Vitamin D.

Serving Size: 4
Prep Time: 0.15

Calories 17	Carbohydrate 3g	Cholesterol 0mg
Protein 2g	Fat 6g	
	% Calories from fat 7%	

VEGETABLES AND VEGETARIAN DISHES

Eggplant Parmesan

- 3 medium eggplants, thinly sliced
- 6 ounces tomato paste
- 1 chopped red bell pepper
- 1 ½ teaspoons oregano
- 1 tablespoon olive oil
- 1 cup mozzarella cheese
- 1 clove crushed garlic
- 1 ½ cups Ricotta cheese
- 2 medium chopped onions
- 1 tablespoon, Parmesan
- 1 pound shredded carrots
- 1 cup chopped parsley
- 1 pound mushrooms
- 1½ cups bread crumbs
- ½ small can black olives, sliced
- 1 teaspoon black pepper
- 1 can (14 ounces) tomatoes

Preheat the oven to 350°F. Sprinkle salt on the eggplant slices and set aside for 20 minutes. Heat the oil in non-stick skillet and sauté the onions and garlic for 3 minutes or until transparent. Add the mushrooms and heat for 2 minutes. Add the shredded carrots and red pepper and cook for 2 minutes more while stirring. Add the tomatoes, tomato paste, olives and oregano. Season to taste and set aside. Drain and wipe dry the eggplant slices. Lay them in a large oiled ovenproof dish and add a layer of mozzarella and ricotta cheese, then a layer of the vegetable mixture. Repeat once more and finally sprinkle with Parmesan cheese. Place in the oven and bake for 45 minutes.

Notes: Excellent source of Vitamin C, A, B6, B1, B2, Folate, Niacin, Calcium, Iron and Zinc.

Serving Size: 8
Prep Time: 1:15 hours

Calories 336	Carbohydrate 48g	Cholesterol 23mg
Protein 19g	Fat 10g	Dietary Fiber 10g
	% Calories from fat 25%	

Fennel Ratatouille

- 2 fennel bulbs
- ½ teaspoon fresh thyme
- 1 pound red ripe tomatoes
- ¼ teaspoon salt
- 2 medium sliced onions
- ¼ teaspoon black pepper
- 2 sliced zucchini
- ½ tablespoon extra virgin olive oil
- 2 tablespoons fresh chopped parsley

Heat the olive oil in a non-stick skillet and sauté the onions for 3-4 minutes until transparent. Add the fennel bulbs cut into slices, layered with zucchini and tomatoes. Sprinkle with herbs and season to taste. Cover the skillet and cook slowly for approximately an hour or until the fennel is tender. Serve hot or cold, garnished with chopped parsley.

Notes: Excellent source of Vitamin C, A and Folate. Good source of Vitamin B6, B1, Niacin, Calcium and Iron.

Serving Size: 4
Prep Time: 1:10 hours

Calories 100	Carbohydrate 19g	Cholesterol 0mg
Protein 4g	Fat 2g	Dietary Fiber 3g
	% Calories from fat 19%	

French Peas

- 2 cups green peas
- ½ cup small white onions
- ½ teaspoon butter (optional)

Boil ½ cup of water and add green peas. Simmer for 5-8 minutes until cooked. Add onions and keep warm with pan covered. Add seasoning to taste. Add butter for optional shiny appearance.

Notes: Excellent source of Vitamin C and Folate. Good source of Vitamin B1.

Serving Size: 4
Prep Time: 0:10

Calories 62	Carbohydrate 11g	Cholesterol 0mg
Protein 4g	Fat <1g	Dietary Fiber 4g
	% Calories from fat 4%	

Frittata with Spinach

- 2 eggs
- ¼ teaspoon red pepper flakes (optional)
- 2 egg whites
- ½ tablespoon extra virgin olive oil
- ½ teaspoon salt
- ½ cup grated Parmesan
- 1 clove garlic
- 1 pound spinach leaves, chopped fine
- 1 teaspoon paprika

Preheat the oven to 350°F. Place the washed spinach in a large saucepan and cook covered for 3-4 minutes, shaking frequently. Drain well. Beat the eggs together (or use 1 ½ cups of liquid egg substitute) and add half of the eggs to the chopped spinach. Mix in 1/4 cup of the grated Parmesan. Prepare an 8 inch round ovenproof dish by lightly brushing with oil. Pour the egg and spinach mixture into the dish and sprinkle with the red pepper flakes. Pour the rest of the egg mixture over this and sprinkle with the rest of the Parmesan and paprika. Bake for 45 minutes and serve hot with a green salad as a main dish.

Notes: Excellent source of Vitamin C, A, B2, Folate, Calcium and Iron. Good source of Zinc.

Serving Size: 4
Prep Time: 1:00 hours

Calories 134	Carbohydrate 5g	Cholesterol 114 mg
Protein 12 g	Fat 7 g	Dietary Fiber 3g
	% Calories from fat 49%	

VEGETABLES AND VEGETARIAN DISHES

Garlic Mashed Potatoes

- 4 peeled potatoes
- 1 teaspoon butter
- ½ cup skim milk
- ¼ teaspoon sea salt
- 3 cloves crushed garlic
- ¼ teaspoon black pepper

Heat the oven to 425°F. Wrap the garlic cloves in aluminum foil and bake for 20 minutes. Unwrap and cool. Slice the potatoes evenly and place in a saucepan. Cover with cold water and bring to a boil. Simmer for 5-8 minutes until soft. Drain and mash until smooth. Cut the base from the garlic cloves and squeeze pulp into mashed potatoes. Warm milk and add to potatoes with butter and seasonings. Serve hot or cold.

Notes: Excellent source of Vitamin C. Good source of Vitamin B6 and Niacin.

Serving Size: 4
Prep Time: 0:30

Calories 111	Carbohydrate 23g	Cholesterol 3mg
Protein 4g	Fat 1g	Dietary Fiber 2g
	% Calories from fat 9%	

Glazed Carrots

    5 medium carrots
    ½ tablespoon fresh lemon juice
    ½ tablespoon butter
    1 tablespoon chopped parsley

Peel and julienne carrots into ¼ inch strips. Place them in a medium saucepan and cover with cold water. Bring to a boil and boil gently for 10-12 minutes or until tender. Drain and set aside in a warm place. In the same pan, melt butter and add lemon juice. Add carrots and toss for 1-2 minutes until well glazed. Serve hot, garnished with fresh chopped parsley.

Notes: Excellent source of Vitamin A. Good source of Vitamin C.

    Serving Size: 4
    Prep Time: 0:30

Calories 52	Carbohydrate 10g	Cholesterol 4mg
Protein 1g	Fat 1g	Dietary Fiber 3g
	% Calories from fat 17%	

Leeks a la Grécque

- 4 medium leeks
- ½ cup rice
- 1 tablespoon olive oil
- 12 small black olives
- 1 cup water
- 1 tablespoon parsley
- 1 tablespoon tomato paste
- 1 teaspoon lemon juice
- 1 teaspoon sugar
- 3 slices lemon

Wash and slice leeks into 1 ½ inch pieces. Steam for 5-6 minutes until cooked. Cool. Boil water, oil, tomato paste and sugar in a large pan and simmer for 5 minutes. Add rice, cover the pot and simmer for 8 minutes or until the liquid is completely absorbed by the rice. Turn off the heat and leave the pan covered for 10 minutes. Add lemon juice and arrange with leeks on a serving dish. Garnish with olives, parsley and lemon slices.

Notes: Excellent source of Vitamin C, B6, B1, Folate and Iron. Good source of Niacin and Calcium.

Serving Size: 4
Prep Time: 0:30

Calories 229	Carbohydrate 48	Cholesterol 0mg
Protein 5g	Fat 5g	Dietary Fiber 3g
	% Calories from fat 19%	

Potatoes au Gratin

- 2 pounds peeled potatoes
- 2 tablespoons Parmesan
- 2 cups skim milk
- ¼ teaspoon salt
- 4 tablespoons Swiss cheese
- ¼ teaspoon white pepper

Place the sliced potatoes in cold water and leave for 5 minutes. Drain and place in an ovenproof gratin dish. Add milk and season to taste with salt and pepper. Cover with foil and place in a medium hot oven (325°F) for 20 minutes. Add grated cheeses and return to the oven for 20-30 minutes or until the potatoes are cooked through. Serve hot.

Notes: Excellent source of Vitamin C, B12 and Calcium. Good source of Vitamin B6 and B2.

Serving Size: 4
Prep Time: 0:30

Calories 111	Carbohydrate 17g	Cholesterol 7mg
Protein 8g	Fat 1g	Dietary Fiber <1g
	% Calories from fat 11%	

VEGETABLES AND VEGETARIAN DISHES

Sautéed Spinach

- 2 pounds fresh washed spinach
- ¼ teaspoon salt
- 1 clove crushed garlic
- ¼ teaspoon black pepper
- 1 tablespoon sesame oil

Place the washed spinach in a large saucepan and cook covered for 3-4 minutes, shaking frequently. Drain well. Heat the sesame oil in a large skillet and add the crushed garlic. Quickly stir-fry the spinach in the garlic and sesame oil and serve hot.

Notes: Excellent source of Vitamin A and Folate. Good source of Vitamin C.

This dish is so low in calories that the % fat calories seems high. The fat source is healthy oils.

Serving Size: 4
Prep Time: 0:10

Calories 38	Carbohydrate 1g	Cholesterol 0mg
Protein <1g	Fat 3g	Dietary Fiber 1g
	% Calories from fat 71%	

Spinach, Brown Rice and Tofu

    1 cup brown rice
    1 tablespoon soy sauce
    ⅔ pound tofu, firm
    1 tablespoon olive oil
    2 pounds spinach leaves
    1 tablespoon sesame seeds

Cook brown rice by covering in cold water with about 1/2 inch extra water on top. Bring to a boil and boil for a minute. Cover, turn the heat down and simmer for 30 - 40 minutes. Check the moisture level twice during cooking and adjust if necessary. Toast the sesame seeds for a few minutes in a medium oven (350° F). Wash and cook spinach in water by shaking a covered pot over a medium heat for 3-5 minutes. Arrange tofu in the middle of an ovenproof dish with spinach around the outside. Moisten with soy sauce and sprinkle the sesame seeds. Warm through in 325° F oven and serve with rice.

Notes: Excellent source of Vitamin C, A, B6, Folate and Iron. Good source of Vitamin B1, B2, Niacin, Calcium and Zinc.

    Serving Size: 4
    Prep Time: 0:45

Calories 164	Carbohydrate 22g	Cholesterol 0mg
Protein 10g	Fat 4g	Dietary Fiber 4g
	% Calories from fat 23%	

Sweet and Sour Vegetables

- 2 cups sliced carrots
- 2 tablespoons tomato paste
- 2 cups chopped bok choy
- ¼ cup soy sauce
- 2 cups chopped green bell pepper
- ⅓ cup pineapple juice
- 3 cups chopped tomatoes
- 1 can sliced water chestnuts
- 1 cup chopped onions
- 1 tablespoon corn starch

Steam the carrots till tender, add the bok choy and green peppers. Set aside. Dissolve the corn starch in the pineapple juice. Place the soy sauce, water and tomato paste in a small pan. Add the corn starch and pineapple mixture and bring to the boil. Stir well until it thickens. Sauté the onions in a covered, heavy-bottomed pan. Add the water chestnuts and the other vegetables and warm through. Add the sauce and serve in a dish with rice or pasta as a main dish.

Notes: Excellent source of Vitamin C, A, B6 and Niacin. Good source of Vitamin B1 and Niacin.

Serving Size: 6
Prep Time: 0:45

Calories 76	Carbohydrate 17g	Cholesterol 0mg
Protein 3g	Fat <1g	Dietary Fiber 4g
	% Calories from fat 6%	

Sweet Potatoes with Almonds

2 pounds sweet potatoes
1 tablespoon slivered almonds

Preheat the oven to 400° F. Toast the slivered almonds for 3-4 minutes until brown. Remove and set aside to cool. Bake the sweet potatoes for 20-30 minutes until soft. (They can also be baked in the microwave oven). When cool, split open and scoop out the center. Mash, adding a little water if necessary. Spread in a serving dish and cover with toasted slivered almonds.

Notes: Excellent source of Vitamin C and A. Good source of Vitamin B6.

Serving Size: 4
Prep Time: 0:30

Calories 82	Carbohydrate 16g	Cholesterol 0mg
Protein 2g	Fat <1g	Dietary Fiber 2g
	% Calories from fat 15%	

VEGETABLES AND VEGETARIAN DISHES

Vegetable Curry

   4   cups brown rice

Sauce
1½ cups cauliflower florets
2   tablespoons olive oil
2   medium carrots, sliced thin
1   tablespoon curry powder
1   cup broccoli florets
2   cloves garlic
1   medium red bell pepper, deseeded and sliced
¼ teaspoon red chili pepper or cayenne
1   medium onion, sliced thin
½ cup vegetable broth
1   cup frozen green peas
2   tablespoons fresh lime juice
1   15 ounce can of tomatoes
1   tablespoon toasted bread crumbs

Cook rice by covering with extra 1/2 inch of water on top. Bring to a boil and boil for a minute uncovered. Cover the pot and simmer gently for 30 minutes. Check water level and adjust so that all water is absorbed and the rice is moist when cooked. Steam the cauliflower, sliced carrots and broccoli for 7-8 minutes, then add the red bell pepper, sliced onion and green peas and steam 3 minutes more. Add the tomatoes at the last minute and mix. Set aside in a casserole dish. Heat oil in a non-stick pan and add curry powder, garlic and red chili pepper. Sauté for 2-3 minutes. Add vegetable broth and boil for 3 minutes. Stir in fresh lime juice and pour over the vegetables. Sprinkle the top with toasted bread crumbs and serve hot.

Notes: Excellent source of Vitamin A, B6, B1, Folate, Niacin and Zinc. Good source of Vitamin B2 and Iron.

Serving Size: 8
Prep Time: 0:30

Calories 434	Carbohydrate 86g	Cholesterol 0mg
Protein 11g	Fat 7g	Dietary Fiber 4g
	% Calories from fat 13%	

Vegetarian Stew

- 1 cup cooked brown rice
- 1 15 ounce can of tomatoes
- ¾ cup bulgur
- 1 can (12 ounces) corn, drained
- ⅔ cup cooked soybeans
- 1 teaspoon olive oil
- ½ pound sliced string beans
- 1 small can green chilies, drained
- 1 teaspoon chili powder
- ½ teaspoon black pepper
- ½ teaspoon hot sauce

Soak the soybeans overnight and discard the water. Cook the brown rice by covering with ½ inch of cold water and bringing to a boil. Reduce heat, cover pot and simmer for 30 minutes or until tender. Cook the bulgur wheat in a similar manner in a separate pot. Drain the cans of chilies and corn. Heat the olive oil and add rice, bulgur, and soybeans. Quickly sauté until well mixed. Add string beans, corn, tomatoes and chilies. Season with chili powder and hot sauce. Add pepper. Simmer for 15 minutes. Serve hot.

Notes: Excellent source of Vitamin C and Folate. Good source of Vitamin A, B6, B1, B2, Niacin and Iron.

Serving Size: 8
Prep Time: 0:45

Calories 210	Carbohydrate 41g	Cholesterol 0mg
Protein 8g	Fat 3g	Dietary Fiber 5g
	% Calories from fat 12%	

VEGETABLES AND VEGETARIAN DISHES

Vegetarian Tofu

1 ½ pounds low-fat tofu, firm
½ teaspoon thyme
½ tablespoon olive oil
¼ teaspoon marjoram
2 cloves crushed garlic
¼ teaspoon savory
2 medium chopped onions
dash Tabasco sauce
1 cup sliced mushrooms
2 cups vegetable broth
⅓ cup Tamari soy sauce
2 cups cooked brown rice
1 teaspoon fresh chopped basil

Heat the olive oil in a non-stick skillet. Add the garlic and onions and sauté for 3-5 minutes until transparent. Add the mushrooms and cook 2 more minutes, shaking the skillet constantly. Remove the vegetables and set aside on a warm dish. Cut the tofu into 1- 1 ½ inch size cubes. In a mixing bowl combine the Tamari, basil, thyme, savory, marjoram and Tabasco. Dip the tofu cubes in the mixture and brown the cubes in the skillet. Add the vegetable broth to the skillet and return the vegetable mixture. Simmer for 10 minutes and serve hot with rice as a main dish.

Notes: Excellent source of Vitamin A and Iron. Good source of Vitamin B6, B1, B2, Folate, Niacin, Calcium and Zinc.

Serving Size: 6
Prep Time: 0:45

Calories 231	Carbohydrate 33g	Cholesterol 1mg
Protein 12g	Fat 6g	Dietary Fiber 3g
	% Calories from fat 23%	

DESSERTS AND COMFORT FOODS

Angel Food Cake

1 ½ cups flour, cake, sifted
¼ teaspoon salt
1 ¾ cups sugar
2 teaspoons vanilla extract
14 egg whites
1 teaspoon fresh lemon juice

Preheat the oven to 300°F. Beat the egg whites (which should be at room temperature) until fluffy but not dry. Fold the sugar with a metal spoon into the egg whites and then lightly fold in the sifted flour. Add the vanilla extract and lemon juice. Pour into an 8 inch diameter cake pan or a 10 inch tube pan. Smooth the top and place in the middle of the oven. Bake until a pale color and the top is spongy. A toothpick should come out clean. Cool in the pan and remove to place on a serving dish by releasing with a palette knife. Serve with fresh fruit and nonfat yogurt or ice cream.

Notes: Good source of Vitamin B1 and B2.

Serves: 10
Prep Time: 0:20
Baking time: 0:30

Calories 219	Carbohydrate 48g	Cholesterol 0mg
Protein 6g	Fat <1g	Dietary Fiber <1g
	% Calories from fat <1%	

DESSERTS AND COMFORT FOODS

Apricot Almond Squares

- 1 cup dried apricot halves
- ½ teaspoon salt
- ½ cup dry roast almonds, ground
- 1 cup flour
- 2 tablespoons butter
- ½ cup egg substitute, liquid
- ¼ cup of oatmeal
- 1 cup light brown sugar
- ¼ cup sugar
- ½ teaspoon baking powder
- 1 teaspoon vanilla extract
- 1 tablespoon confectioner's sugar
- ½ teaspoon almond extract

Preheat the oven to 350°F. Place apricots in a pan of cold water and bring to a boil. Cover and simmer for 6-8 minutes. Drain and pat dry. Slice thinly, cover and set aside. Blend the butter and oatmeal with 2 tablespoons water. Mix in half of the flour and the ground almonds with a metal spoon. Spread over the bottom of a 9 inch baking pan. Bake for 20 minutes. While the pastry is baking, sift the rest of the flour with the baking powder and salt. Lightly beat the egg substitute with the brown sugar and blend in the flour mixture. Add the vanilla and almond extracts and stir in the apricots. Spread over the pastry. Bake for 30 minutes until brown. Cool and sift confectioner's sugar over the squares before serving.

Serves: 36
Prep Time: 0:10
Baking time: 0:50

Calories 67	Carbohydrate 13g	Cholesterol 0mg
Protein 1g	Fat 1g Dietary Fiber 1g	% Calories from fat 15%

DESSERTS AND COMFORT FOODS

Apricot and Strawberry Cake

- 2 ¾ cups flour
- 2 eggs, beaten
- 2 ½ teaspoons baking powder
- 1 ½ teaspoons vanilla
- 1 ¾ cups sugar
- 9 tablespoons strawberry jam
- 1 ¼ cups skim milk
- 8 large strawberries, sliced thin
- ¾ cup apricots, puréed
- 2 tablespoons apricot brandy glaze

Preheat the oven to 375°F. Sift the flour, baking powder and sugar in a mixing bowl and stir to blend. Using a metal spoon combine the skim milk, apricot purée, eggs and vanilla with the dry ingredients. Pour the batter into two 8" cake pans sprayed with oil. Bake for 25 - 30 minutes or until a toothpick comes out dry from the center. Let the cake cool in the pan for 5 minutes before removing and cooling on a rack. Split each cake in half horizontally and fill with strawberry preserves. Brush the apricot brandy glaze (or apricot glaze) on the top and arrange strawberry slices in a petal-shaped pattern on the top. Glaze the strawberry slices also and serve with fresh whipped cream; low or nonfat yogurt or ice cream.

Notes: Excellent source of Vitamin C, B1 and B2. Good source of Vitamin A, Folate, Niacin, Calcium and Iron. Good source of Vitamin A, B6 and Zinc.

Serves: 8
Prep Time: 0:10
Baking time: 0:35

Calories 465	Carbohydrate 106g	Cholesterol 54mg
Protein 9g	Fat 2g	Dietary Fiber 4g
	% Calories from fat 4%	

DESSERTS AND COMFORT FOODS

Banana Bread

- 2 medium bananas
- 1 tablespoon honey
- 3 egg whites
- 1 ½ cups flour
- 2 tablespoons canola oil
- 2 teaspoons baking powder
- ½ teaspoon cinnamon
- ½ teaspoon salt
- ½ teaspoon nutmeg

Preheat the oven to 350°F. Lightly grease a 9 X 5 inch loaf pan. Beat the egg whites until fluffy, but not dry. Mash the bananas with the honey and canola oil and fold into the egg whites. In another bowl, sift the flour and salt. Add the baking powder, ground cinnamon and ground nutmeg. Combine with the banana mixture using light, firm strokes. Place the batter into the loaf pan and bake for 50 to 60 minutes or until a toothpick comes out clean. Cool for 10 minutes before turning out. Slice and serve warm or cold.

Notes: Good source of Vitamin B1 & B6, Thiamin, Riboflavin and Folate

Variations: Add 8 apricot halves, finely chopped OR 1/2 cups golden raisins OR 1/3 cup pecans or English walnuts, chopped.

Serves: 4
Prep Time: 0:10
Baking time: 1:00

Calories 327	Carbohydrate 58g	Cholesterol 0mg
Protein 8g	Fat 8g	Dietary Fiber 3g
	% Calories from fat 22%	

Ginger Cookies

½ cup apple sauce
1 ¼ teaspoons baking soda
8 ounces butter (2 ½ cup sticks)
10 ½ teaspoons cinnamon
1 ¾ cups sugar
2 tablespoons ginger
¾ cup brown sugar
1 tablespoon cloves
1 medium egg
1 tablespoon nutmeg
⅓ cup molasses
½ teaspoon salt
2 ¾ cups white flour
½ cup powdered sugar

Preheat the oven to 350ºF. Cream butter and sugar together until light and fluffy, taking about 8 to 10 minutes by hand or 4 to 5 minutes in a food processor. Lightly fold in the beaten egg and molasses. Sift flour, baking soda and salt and lightly fold into the mixture with firm strokes using a metal spoon. Season with the cinnamon, ginger, cloves, nutmeg and salt. Form ¾ inch round balls of dough, flatten a little and dip the top into ½ cup of powdered sugar. Place on a non-stick cookie sheet with the sugar side up. Bake for 12 to 15 minutes depending upon how crisp you like them. Serve warm.

Serves: 36
Prep Time: 0:20

Calories 151	Carbohydrate 26g	Cholesterol 19 mg
Protein 1g	Fat 5g	Dietary Fiber 1g
	% Calories from fat 30%	

DESSERTS AND COMFORT FOODS

Ice Cream Base

- 1 tablespoon corn starch
- ½ cup honey or sugar
- 2 cups milk
- 2 egg yolks
- 2 cups Greek style yogurt

Heat 1 ½ cups of milk over a double boiler or in a glass bowl over water that is almost boiling. Add cornstarch mixed with the remaining half cup of milk and incorporate into the milk by gently stirring over the heat. Add egg yolks and continue to stir for about 2 minutes until the mixture is thickened. Remove from the heat and allow to cool. Once cold, stir in the cream and any fruit and other flavorings the add to an ice cream maker or place in the freezer and stir every twenty minutes. Yields 3 cups of ice cream.

Nutritional Analysis of Ice cream base (add about 80 calories for fruit puree)

Serves: 6
Prep Time: 3:00

Calories 201	Carbohydrate 37g	Cholesterol 78 mg
Protein 6 g	Fat 4 g	Dietary Fiber 0g
	% Calories from fat 18%	

Key Lime Pie

- 1 cup Graham cracker crumbs
- ½ cup sugar
- 2 tablespoons unsalted butter
- ½ teaspoon vanilla extract
- 1 tablespoon water
- 2 cups nonfat yogurt
- 1 packet gelatin powder
- 1 tablespoon lime rind
- 6 tablespoons fresh lime juice

Mix the Graham cracker crumbs with the butter and line an 8 inch baking pan. Dissolve the gelatin powder in the water and add the lime juice and sugar. Heat in a small saucepan until the sugar is dissolved. Allow to cool and add the yogurt and fresh grated lime rind. When beginning to thicken, place on top of the crumbs and leave to set. Garnish with sugared fresh lime or lemon rind. Serve chilled.

Notes: Good source of Vitamin C, B2 and Calcium.

Serves: 6
Prep Time: 0:20
Stand Time: 1:00

Calories 253	Carbohydrate 35g	Cholesterol 12mg
Protein 18g	Fat 6g	Dietary Fiber 1g
	% Calories from fat 19%	

DESSERTS AND COMFORT FOODS

Peanut Butter Sesame Seed Bars

- ½ cup vanilla protein powder
- ½ cup honey
- ¾ cup skim dry milk
- 2 tablespoons warm water
- 1 cup dry oatmeal flakes
- 2 tablespoons sesame seeds
- ¾ cup low-fat peanut butter

Combine all of the ingredients in a mixing bowl. Spray a 9 X 9 baking pan with oil and press the mixture into the pan. Refrigerate for at least 30 minutes before cutting into brownie shaped bars.

Notes: Excellent source of Vitamin B6, B1, B2, Folate, Niacin and Zinc. Good source of Vitamin A, Calcium and Iron.

Serves: 12
Prep Time: 0:05
Stand Time: 0:30

Calories 143	Carbohydrate 25g	Cholesterol 1mg
Protein 9g	Fat 2g	Dietary Fiber 2g
	% Calories from fat 9%	

DESSERTS AND COMFORT FOODS

Cinnamon Apple Sauce

    2 cups apple sauce
    1 teaspoon cinnamon

For homemade apple sauce, wash, peel and core 1 pound of apples. Add piece of lemon and cook over low heat until soft. Blend and sweeten to taste. Add cinnamon. Notes: Jarred apple sauce may also be used for a quick and easy dessert. Baby food is useful for single servings.

Good source of Vitamin C

Serving Size: 4
Prep Time: 0:20

Calories 68	Carbohydrate 18g	Cholesterol 0mg
Protein <1g	Fat <1g	Dietary Fiber 3g
	% Calories from fat 6%	

DESSERTS AND COMFORT FOODS

Pineapple Meringue

    1 cup pineapple chunks, light syrup
    1 egg yolk
    1 cup pineapple juice
    ½ cup sugar
    1 tablespoon butter
    2 egg whites
    1 tablespoon flour

Preheat the oven to 350°F. Drain the pineapple chunks and retain the light syrup. Melt the butter in a saucepan and add the flour. Stir over a gentle heat for 2-3 minutes until a roux forms and the mixture comes away from the sides easily. Add the syrup and pineapple juice (total of one cup) and bring to a boil, stirring all the time. When the sauce is thickened, add the egg yolk and all of the pineapple chunks except one or two for decoration. Remove from the heat and pour into a greased 9" pie dish. Beat the egg whites until fluffy but not dry. Fold in the sugar and continue to beat until shiny and stiff. Spoon over the pineapple mixture and garnish with the left over pineapple chunks. Place in the oven for 3-4 minutes until the top has browned. Serve hot.

Note: Excellent source of Vitamin C.

Serves: 4
Prep Time: 0:20

Calories 146	Carbohydrate 29g	Cholesterol 41mg
Protein 2.1g	Fat 3g	Dietary Fiber 1g
	% Calories from fat 18%	

Fresh Fruit Salad

- 1 apple, peeled and chopped
- 1 nectarine, chopped
- 8 small seedless grapes, peeled
- ½ banana, peeled and sliced
- 1 can mandarin oranges, light syrup
- 1 pear, peeled and chopped
- 1 plum, chopped
- 2 tablespoons lemon juice

Combine all of the ingredients in a mixing bowl. Chill in the refrigerator for at least one hour. Transfer to individual dessert dishes and serve garnished with tiny sprigs of mint or borage.

Notes: Excellent source of Vitamin C, A, B6 and Iron. Good source of Vitamin B1, B2 and Folate.

Serves: 4
Prep Time: 0:20
Stand Time: 1:00

Calories 320	Carbohydrate 82g	Cholesterol 0mg
Protein 4g	Fat 1g	Dietary Fiber 8g
	% Calories from fat 3%	

DESSERTS AND COMFORT FOODS

Fresh Peaches in Lemon Juice

- 6 fresh peaches, peeled and sliced
- 2 lemons, juiced
- 2 tablespoons sugar

Arrange peach slices in a serving dish and cover with the sugar and lemon juice. Leave for at least 2 hours in the refrigerator. The peaches will leach juice into the lemon juice and create a sweet sauce with the sugar. This is best served at room temperature after a main course of meat to cleanse the palate.

Notes: Excellent source of Vitamin C. Good source of Vitamin A.

Serves: 4
Prep Time: 0:05
Stand Time: 2:00

Calories 91	Carbohydrate 26g	Cholesterol 0g
Protein 2g	Fat <1g	Dietary Fiber 3g
	% Calories from fat 2%	

DESSERTS AND COMFORT FOODS

Pears in Red Wine

- 4 pears
- ½ teaspoon cinnamon
- 3 cups red wine
- 1 cup water
- ¾ cup sugar
- 2 tablespoons fresh lemon juice

Peel and core the pears. Cover with cold water and add the lemon juice to prevent them from turning brown. In a large saucepan place the red wine, sugar, cinnamon and water. Heat the mixture until the sugar is dissolved. Add the pears and simmer gently for 10-15 minutes until soft, turning them so they are evenly colored by the wine. Remove the pears when soft and place in a serving dish. Bring to the liquid to a boil and reduce by half. Coat the pears with the sauce and serve warm.

Notes: Good source of Vitamin C.

Serves: 4
Prep Time: 0:20

Calories 373	Carbohydrate 66g	Cholesterol 0mg
Protein 1g	Fat 1g	Dietary Fiber 4
	% Calories from fat 2%	

DESSERTS AND COMFORT FOODS

Strawberry Delight

- 1 packet gelatin powder, dissolved in water
- 1 cup low fat yogurt with fruit
- ½ cup fresh sliced strawberries

Prepare the gelatin according to the instructions. When it begins to set, stir in the yogurt and strawberries. Pour into individual dessert dishes and refrigerate until set. Garnish with fresh strawberries and whipped cream.

Notes: Excellent source of Calcium.

Serves: 4
Prep Time: 0:15
Standing Time: 2:00

Calories 143	Carbohydrate 31g	Cholesterol 3mg
Protein 4g	Fat <1g	Dietary Fiber <1g
	% Calories from fat 5%	

Rhubarb and Cinnamon Flan

- 1 cup Graham cracker crumbs
- 2 tablespoons flour
- 2 tablespoons unsalted butter
- ½ teaspoon cinnamon
- 1 pound fresh rhubarb
- 2 tablespoons cream cheese
- ¼ cup sugar
- 1 tablespoon sour cream

Combine Graham cracker crumbs with melted butter and line 8 inch baking pan. Prepare rhubarb by washing, removing any blemished or coarse parts and then slicing and cutting into 1/2 inch pieces. Place rhubarb in pie crust. Mix sugar, flour, cream cheese and cinnamon and then spoon over the rhubarb. Bake in pre-heated oven at 425 for 30 minutes. Allow to cool and serve with fresh, whipped cream garnished with a little cinnamon.

Serves: 6
Prep Time: 0:10
Baking Time: 0:30

Calories 166	Carbohydrate 25g	Cholesterol 14 mg
Protein 3 g	Fat 7 g	Dietary Fiber 2 g
	% Calories from fat 38%	

BEVERAGES AND SMOOTHIES

Aloha Delight

    1 cup skim milk
    ½ teaspoon pineapple extract
    2 tablespoons vanilla protein powder
    1 tablespoon orange juice
    ½ teaspoon coconut extract
    3 ice cubes

Combine ingredients in a blender and blend until smooth. Serve chilled, garnished with fresh pineapple and a sprig of mint.

Notes: Excellent source of Vitamin C, B1, B2, Calcium and Iron. Good source of Vitamin A and B6.

    Serves: 1
    Prep Time: 0:05

Calories 186	Carbohydrate 24g	Cholesterol 4mg
Protein 17g	Fat 1g	Dietary Fiber 3g
	% Calories from fat 6%	

Apple Pie Smoothie

    2 tablespoons vanilla protein powder
    ½ teaspoon cinnamon
    ¼ cup apples
    1 cup skim milk
    1 dash nutmeg
    3 ice cubes

Blend all ingredients together and serve chilled.

Notes: Excellent source of Vitamin C, B6, B12, B1, B2, Folate, Calcium, Iron and Zinc. Good source of Vitamin A.

    Serves: 1
    Prep Time: 0:10

Calories 184	Carbohydrate 27g	Cholesterol 4mg
Protein 16g	Fat 1g	Dietary Fiber 4g
	% Calories from fat 6%	

BEVERAGES AND SMOOTHIES

Banana Fruit Smoothie

- 2 tablespoons vanilla protein powder
- ½ cup frozen peaches
- 4 ounces nonfat yogurt
- ½ medium banana
- 4 fluid ounces water
- 3 ice cubes

Blend all ingredients and serve chilled, garnished with a slice of banana.

Notes: Excellent source of Vitamin C, B6, B1, B2, Iron and Zinc. Good source of Calcium.

Serves: 1
Prep Time: 0:05

Calories 310	Carbohydrate 62g	Cholesterol 2mg
Protein 16g	Fat 1g	Dietary Fiber 6g
	% Calories from fat 3%	

Black Forest Smoothie

- 2 tablespoons chocolate protein powder
- ½ banana
- ½ teaspoon black walnut extract
- 4 ice cubes
- 8 fluid ounces skim milk

Combine ingredients in a blender and serve chilled garnished with chocolate sprinkles.

Notes: Excellent source of Vitamin C, B6, B12, B1, B2, Calcium and Zinc. Good source of Vitamin A and Iron.

Serves: 1
Prep Time: 0:05

Calories 175	Carbohydrate 26g	Cholesterol 9mg
Protein 16g	Fat 1g	Dietary Fiber 16g
	% Calories from fat 5%	

BEVERAGES AND SMOOTHIES

Cappuccino Smoothie

- 2 tablespoons chocolate protein powder
- 4 ounces vanilla frozen yogurt
- 3 ice cubes
- 4 fluid ounces skim milk
- 1 tablespoon instant coffee

Place all ingredients in a blender and mix until smooth.

Notes: Excellent source of Vitamin B12, B2 and Calcium.

Serves: 1
Prep Time: 0:05

Calories 196	Carbohydrate 28g	Cholesterol 4mg
Protein 19g	Fat 1g	Dietary Fiber 0g
	% Calories from fat 4%	

Extra Chocolatey Smoothie

- 1 cup skim milk
- 1 teaspoon Hershey's cocoa
- 2 tablespoons chocolate protein powder
- ¼ teaspoon vanilla extract
- ¼ teaspoon chocolate syrup
- 3 ice cubes

Combine all the ingredients in a blender and blend until smooth.
Serve chilled, garnished with chocolate sprinkles.

Notes: Excellent source of Vitamin B12, B2 and Calcium. Good source of Vitamin A.
Optional addition: 1 teaspoon instant coffee.

Serves: 1
Prep Time: 0:05

Calories 212	Carbohydrate 17g	Cholesterol 70mg
Protein 32g	Fat 2g	Dietary Fiber 2g
	% Calories from fat <1%	

BEVERAGES AND SMOOTHIES

Fruit-Juicy Smoothie

- 2 tablespoons berry protein powder
- 4 strawberries
- 8 fluid ounces cranberry juice
- 3 ice cubes

Combine ingredients in a blender and serve chilled, garnished with a strawberry.

Notes: Excellent source of Vitamin C, B6, B1, B2, Iron and Zinc. Good source of Calcium.

Serves: 1
Prep Time: 0:05

Calories 125	Carbohydrate 21g	Cholesterol 0mg
Protein 8g	Fat 1g	Dietary Fiber 3g
	% Calories from fat 7%	

BEVERAGES AND SMOOTHIES

Kiwi Quencher

- 2 tablespoons vanilla protein powder
- ½ banana
- 8 fluid ounces water
- 3 ice cubes
- 1 kiwi fruit
- 2 drops green chartreuse

Combine ingredients in a blender. Serve chilled with a slice of kiwi fruit as garnish.

Notes: Excellent source of Vitamin C, B6, B2, Iron and Zinc. Good source of Vitamin B1.

Serves: 1
Prep Time: 0:05

Calories 80	Carbohydrate 10g	Cholesterol 0mg
Protein 8g	Fat <1g	Dietary Fiber 3g
	% Calories from fat 7%	

Mango Special

- 2 cups mangos diced
- ¼ cup lemon juice
- 2 cups orange juice
- 2 cups water
- 2 tablespoons sugar
- 3 ice cubes
- ¼ cup lime juice

Combine the ingredients in a blender. Strain and serve in a pitcher either for breakfast or as a non-alcoholic cocktail. This is excellent with champagne.

Notes: Excellent source of Vitamin C and A. Good source of Folate.

Serves: 8
Prep Time: 0:10

Calories 70	Carbohydrate 18g	Cholesterol 0mg
Protein 1g	Fat 3g	Dietary Fiber 1g
	% Calories from Fat 3%	

Orange Blossom Smoothie

- 2 tablespoons vanilla protein powder
- ½ orange
- ½ teaspoon orange extract
- 3 ice cubes
- 8 fluid ounces skim milk

Combine ingredients in a blender and serve chilled, garnished with a slice of orange.

Notes: Excellent source of Vitamin C, B6, B12, B1, B2, Calcium, Iron and Zinc. Good source of Vitamin A.

Serves: 1
Prep Time: 0:05

Calories 168	Carbohydrate 22g	Cholesterol 4mg
Protein 16g	Fat 1g	Dietary Fiber 3g
	% Calories from fat 6%	

Passionate Papaya Smoothie

- 2 tablespoons vanilla protein powder
- 8 fluid ounces apple juice
- ½ papaya
- 1 dash cinnamon

Blend together and serve chilled.

Notes: Excellent source of Vitamin C, B6, B1, B2, Folate, Iron and Zinc. Good source of Vitamin A.

Serves: 1
Prep Time: 0:05

Calories 256	Carbohydrate 54g	Cholesterol 0mg
Protein 10g	Fat 1g	Dietary Fiber 6g
	% Calories from fat 4%	

Peach Milk Smoothie

- 2 tablespoons vanilla protein powder
- ½ fresh peach
- 8 fluid ounces skim milk
- 3 ice cubes
- 1 teaspoon peach brandy extract (optional)

Combine ingredients in a blender and serve chilled, garnished with a slice of peach.

Notes: Excellent source of Vitamin C, B6, B12, B1, B2, Calcium, Iron and Zinc. Good source of Vitamin A.

Serves: 1
Prep Time: 0:05

Calories 165	Carbohydrate 22g	Cholesterol 4mg
Protein 16g	Fat 1g	Dietary Fiber 3g
	% Calories from fat 6%	

BEVERAGES AND SMOOTHIES

Prune Smoothie

- 2 tablespoons vanilla protein powder
- 8 fluid ounces prune juice

Blend. Serve chilled.

Notes: Excellent source of Vitamin C, B6, B1, B2, Iron and Zinc. Good source of Niacin.

Serves: 1
Prep Time: 0:05

Calories 216	Carbohydrate 44g	Cholesterol 0mg
Protein 9g	Fat 1g	Dietary Fiber 4g
	% Calories from fat 3%	

Raspberry RazMaTaz

- 2 tablespoons chocolate protein powder
- ½ banana
- 8 fluid ounces water
- 3 ice cubes
- ⅓ cup raspberries, fresh or frozen

Combine all ingredients in a blender. Serve chilled, garnished with fresh raspberries and a sprig of mint.

Notes: Excellent source of Vitamin C and Folate.

Serves: 1
Prep Time: 0:05

Calories 162	Carbohydrate 32g	Cholesterol 5mg
Protein 9g	Fat <1g	Dietary Fiber 7g
	% Calories from fat 5%	

BEVERAGES AND SMOOTHIES

Soda Fountain Shake

- 2 tablespoons vanilla protein powder
- ½ banana
- 5 fluid ounces skim milk
- 3 ice cubes
- 3 fluid ounces seltzer water

Blend together and serve chilled. Banana may be substituted with peach. Garnish with a slice of banana.

Notes: Excellent source of Vitamin C, B6, B1, B2, Calcium, Iron and Zinc.

Serves: 1
Prep Time: 0:05

Calories 133	Carbohydrate 18g	Cholesterol 2mg
Protein 13g	Fat 1g	Dietary Fiber 3g
	% Calories from fat 6%	

Spicy Tomato Juice

- 2 cups tomato juice
- 2 stalks celery
- 1 teaspoon Tabasco sauce
- 1 pinch salt
- 1 teaspoon fresh lemon juice
- 1 pinch sugar

Combine all the ingredients in a jug. Chill for 30 minutes and serve garnished with celery stalks.

Notes: Excellent source of Vitamin A, C, Folate. Good source of Vitamin B1 and Niacin.

Serves: 2
Prep Time: 0:10

Calories 133	Carbohydrate 18g	Cholesterol 0mg
Protein 13g	Fat 1g	Dietary Fiber 3g
	% Calories from fat 6%	

BEVERAGES AND SMOOTHIES

Strawberry Daiquiri

- 6 fluid ounces rum
- 4 cups strawberries
- ½ cup fresh lime juice
- 6 ice cubes
- 2 tablespoons sugar

Combine rum, lime juice, sugar and ice cubes in a blender. Add the strawberries after the sugar has dissolved and continue to blend at high speed until the mixture is smooth. Serve with sugar around the rim of each glass.

Notes: Excellent source of Vitamin C. Good source of Folate.

Serves: 4
Prep Time: 0:10

Calories 173	Carbohydrate 20g	Cholesterol 0mg
Protein 1g	Fat 1g	Dietary Fiber 4g
	% Calories from fat 6%	

Strawberry Sensation

- 2 tablespoons strawberry protein powder
- 8 fluid ounces water
- 1 apricot
- 1 cup strawberries
- 3 ice cubes

Combine all ingredients in a blender. Garnish with a strawberry and sprig of fresh mint.

Notes: Excellent source of Vitamin C, B6, B1, B2, Iron and Zinc. Good source of Folate and Calcium.

Serves: 1
Prep Time: 0:05

Calories 124	Carbohydrate 21g	Cholesterol 0mg
Protein 9g	Fat 2g	Dietary Fiber 6g
	% Calories from fat 11%	

BEVERAGES AND SMOOTHIES

Vanilla Smoothie

    2   tablespoons vanilla protein powder
    3   ice cubes
    6   fluid ounces skim milk
    4   ounces nonfat yogurt

Blend all ingredients together. Serve chilled, garnished with fresh fruit.

Notes: Excellent source of Vitamin B6, B12, B2, Calcium and Zinc. Good source of Vitamin C, B1 and Iron.

    Serves: 1
    Prep Time: 0:05

Calories 228	Carbohydrate 31g	Cholesterol 6mg
Protein 23g	Fat 1g	Dietary Fiber 3g
	% Calories from fat 5%	

Wild Berry-Orange Smoothie

- 2 tablespoons berry protein powder
- 4 strawberries
- 8 fluid ounces orange juice
- 3 ice cubes

Combine all ingredients in a blender and serve chilled, garnished with a fresh strawberry.

Notes: Excellent source of Vitamin C, B6, B1, B2, Folate, Iron and Zinc. Good source of Vitamin A and Calcium.

Serves: 1
Prep Time: 0:05

Calories 192	Carbohydrate 36g	Cholesterol 0mg
Protein 10g	Fat 2g	Dietary Fiber 3g
	% Calories from fat 7%	

RECIPE INDEX

Appetizers
- Babaghanoush 33
- Bean Dip 34
- Bruschetta 35
- Chicken Liver Pâté 36
- Curry Dip 37
- Guacamole 38

Soups and Broths
- Beef (or veal) Stock 39
- Chicken Broth 40
- Chicken and Okra Gumbo 41
- Chicken Soup 42
- Gazpacho 43
- Green Pea Soup 44
- Immuno-Soup 45
- Minestrone 46
- Miso 47
- Phytomineral Soup 48
- Rice and Celery Soup 49
- Root Vegetable Soup 50
- Tomato Soup 51

Beans, Pasta and Rice
- Adzuki Beans and Rice 52
- Baked Beans 53
- Bean, Noodle and Nut Casserole 54
- Blackeyed Peas 55
- Brown Rice Pilaf 56
- Flageolets (Small French Green Beans) ... 57
- Lemon Rice 58

Beans, Pasta and Rice, Cont.
- Lentil and Pecan Casserole 59
- Lentil Patties 60
- Mexican Bean Pie 61
- Navy Bean Stew 62
- Noodles with Tuna 63
- Pasta and Eggplant 64
- Pasta Primavera 65
- Quinoa-Nut Vegetable Pilaf 66
- Risotto 67
- Spaghetti with Artichoke Hearts 68
- Southern Style Beans and Rice 69
- Stir-fry Vegetables and Rice 70
- Tasty Rice and Tofu 71

Fish
- Baked Red Snapper 72
- Baked Salmon 73
- Barbecued Fish with Tarragon Sauce 74
- Broiled Orange Roughy 75
- Creamy Dijon Sole 76
- Ginger-Sesame Salmon 77
- Grilled Tuna 78
- Halibut with Broccoli and Almonds 79
- Monkfish, Mushrooms and Lentils 80
- Sea Bass with Apples 81
- Sizzling Swordfish, Broccoli & Peanuts ... 82
- Teriyaki Salmon 83
- Trout with Almonds 84
- White Fish with Ginger and Lemon 85

Chicken

- Chicken Curry 86
- Chicken in Soy Sauce 87
- Chicken with Tarragon 88
- Lemon Chicken and English Walnuts 89
- Oven-baked Sesame Chicken 90

Vegetables and Vegetarian Dishes

- Brussels sprouts and Chestnuts 91
- Collard Greens with Pinenuts................. 92
- Creamed Spinach 93
- Eggplant Parmesan 94
- Fennel Ratatouille............................. 95
- French Peas 96
- Frittata with Spinach 97
- Garlic Mashed Potatoes........................ 98
- Glazed Carrots 99
- Leeks a la Grécque............................ 100
- Potatoes au Gratin 101
- Sautéed Spinach 102
- Spinach, Brown Rice and Tofu 103
- Sweet and Sour Vegetables 104
- Sweet Potatoes with Almonds 105
- Vegetable Curry 106
- Vegetarian Stew 107
- Vegetarian Tofu 108

Desserts and Comfort Foods

- Angel Food Cake 109
- Apricot Almond Squares 110
- Apricot and Strawberry Cake................ 111
- Banana Bread 112
- Ginger Cookies 113

Desserts and Comfort Foods, cont.

- Ice Cream Base 114
- Key Lime Pie 115
- Peanut Butter Sesame Seed Bars 116
- Cinnamon Apple Sauce 117
- Pineapple Meringue 118
- Fresh Fruit Salad 119
- Fresh Peaches in Lemon Juice 120
- Pears in Red Wine 121
- Strawberry Delight 122
- Rhubarb and Cinnamon Flan................ 123

Beverages and Smoothies

- Aloha Delight.................................. 124
- Apple Pie Smoothie 125
- Banana Fruit Smoothie 126
- Black Forest Smoothie....................... 127
- Cappuccino Smoothie........................ 128
- Extra Chocolatey Smoothie 129
- Fruit-Juicy Smoothie......................... 130
- Kiwi Quencher 131
- Mango Special................................. 132
- Orange Blossom Smoothie................... 133
- Passionate Papaya Smoothie................ 134
- Peach Milk Smoothie 135
- Prune Smoothie 136
- Raspberry RazMaTaz 137
- Soda Fountain Shake......................... 138
- Spicy Tomato Juice........................... 139
- Strawberry Daiquiri 140
- Strawberry Sensation 141
- Vanilla Smoothie.............................. 142
- Wild Berry-Orange Smoothie 143

HANDBOOK TEXT INDEX

Abraxane 12
Accutane 12
Acorn squash.. 21
Abdominal discomfort 6,27
Adriamycin 12
Adrucil.. 12
Afinitor 12
Alcohol consumption 2,4,9,12-18,22,24
Alemtuzumab.. 12
Alimta... 12
Alkeran 12
Alpha Lipoic Acid 19-22
Anastrozole 12
Antioxidants 2-3,6-7,19-21,24,38
Appetite 20,24,31
Apricots................... 4,23,24,27,110,111
Arimidex... 12
Aromasin 12
Arranon 12
Arsenic trioxide 17
Arzerra.. 12
Asparaginase... 13
Asparagus 21, 25 30, 65
ATRA.. 17
Avastin.. 12
Avocado 2, 10, 12-18, 21-22, 25-26, 29, 38
B vitamins..................... 2,3,7,12,13,15,18
BAN.. 13
BCG 17
Bell peppers 4,61,65
Bendamustine 17
Beta carotene 3,4,19,24

Bevacizumab... 12
Bexarotene.. 16
Bexxar 13
Bicalutamide... 13
BCNU 13
BiCNU 13
Bitter melon 21
Black currants 21
Blackberries 21
Black Raspberries 2,21
Blenoxane 13
Bleomycin 13
Blueberries 2,4,21,25,30
Body Mass Index (BMI)............................. 5
Body weight 5-8, 22
Borage 8,26,119
Bortezomib... 17
Broccoli 3,12-16,27,29,79,82,106
Busulfan 13
Busulfex 13
BZM.. 17
Cabazitaxel 15
Caffeine 12-13,16-17
Campath.. 13
Camptosar... 13
Cantaloupe 4,21,24
Carbohydrates 27
Carboplatin 13
Carmustine.. 13
Casodex.. 13
CeeNU 13
Cerubine.. 13

Cetuximab	11,13
Chemotherapy	8-11,19-20,22,27
Chewing difficulties	22
Chlorambucil	15
Cisplatin	13
Cladribine	15
CMF	18
Coenzyme Q10	21,22
Constipation	10,12,16,17,22,23,28
coumadin	18
Cruciferous vegetable family	3,21
Curcumin	13-15
Cyclophosphamide	13,15
Cytarabine	13
Cytosine arabinoside	13
Cytoxan	13
Dacarbazine	11,13
Dairy products	2,5-6,12,14-15,19
Dasatinib	16
Daunorubicin	13
Decadron	18
Deltasone	18
DepoCyt	13
Dexamethasone	18
Dexrazoxane	18
Diarrhea	6,12,14-17,19,22,23,28
Digestive enzymes	6,9,27
Docetaxel	16
DITC-Dome	13
Doxil	13
Doxorubicin liposomal	13
Efudex	13
Ellence	13
Eloxatin	13
Elspar	13
Energy	5,6,8,20,24,26
Ephedra	21
Epirubicin chloride	13
Epogen	18
Epoetin alfa	18
Erbitux	13
Eribulin mesylate	14
Erlotinib	16
Essential fatty acids	12
Etoposide	17
Eulexin	14
Everolimus	12
Evista	14
Exemestane	12
Expedient Diet	6,12
Fareston	14
Faslodex	14
Fats	6,22,26,27
Femara	14
Fish oil	8
Flaxseed	14,23,26
Fluorouracil	13
Fludarabine	14
Fludara-IV	14
Fluorouracil	13
Flutamide	15
Folic Acid/folate	15,18,25
Folinic acid	18
FOLFOX	19
Folotyn	15
5-FU	14
Fulvestrant	15
GM-CSF	15
Gamma Linoleic Acid (GLA)	26
Garlic	3,19,21,23,25,28,29,32,35,38,39, 41-43,45,46,48-50,52,55-57,60-62, 64,66-68,71,72,75,77,79,80,82, 85-88,90,92,94,97,98,102,106
Gefitinib	14

Gemcitabine	14
Gemtuzumab	14
Gemzar	14
Ginseng	8,21
Gleevec	14
Gliadel	14
Glutathione	12,19
goseretin	18
Grapes	2,4,7,21,25,119
Green tea	8,14,19,21
Halaven	14
Hematinic supplements	19
Herbs	7-9,19,21,25,74,95
Herceptin	14
Hycamtin	14
Hydrea	14
Hydroxyurea	14
Ibritumomab tiuxetan	17
Idamycin	14
Idarubicin	14
Ifex	14
Ifosfamide	14
Immunity	22,24
Interferon	16,18
Intron A	18
Iressa	14
Irinotecan	13
Iron	9,18,25,30,36,38,42,44-46,48-49,51-57, 59,60-69,71,73-75,77,79,80-85,88,94,95, 97,100,103,106,107,108,111,116,119, 124-127,130,131,133-136,138,141-143
Isotretinoin	12
Ixabepilone	15
Ixempra	15
Jevtana	15
Kava	21
Lapatinib	17
Lenalidomide	16
Lemon	3,4,10,18,28,29,33,37,38,43,58, 63,74,77,84,85,89,93,99,100,109, 117,119,120,121,132,139
Leukine	15
Leukovorin	18
Leuprolide	15,17
Leustatin	15
Lime	4,11,29,106,115,132,140
Liposomal Ara-C	13
Lomustine	12
L-PAM	12
Lupron	15
Lycopene	4,25,35
Magnesium	2,12,13,14,16,18,25,30
Manganese	25
Matulane	15
Meal replacement drinks	19,22,24
Mechlorethamine	15
Megace/megasterol	18
Melphalan	12
Mercaptopurine	15
Mesna	15,18
Mesnex	15,18
Methotrexate	11,17
Meticorten	18
Mexate	17
Milk Thistle	19,20,22
Mitomycin	15
Mitoxantrone	15
MTC	15
Mustargen	15
Mutamycin	15
Myleran	13
Mylocel	15
N-acetyl cysteine (NAC)	20
Nausea	12,13,17,22-23
Navelbine	15

Nelarabine	12
Neosar	15
Neulasta	18
Neumega	18
Neupogen	18
Nexavar	15
Nilandron	15
Nilotinib	16
Nilutamide	15
Nipent	15
Nolvadex	16
Novantrone	15
Octreotide	16
Ofatumumab	12
Omega-3 fatty acids	3,9,26
Oncovin	15
oprevelkin	18
Oxaliplatin	13
Paclitaxel	12,16
Panitumumab	17
Pantothenic Acid	25
Parsley	11,21,29,33,36,42,45,48, 49,50,57,58,62,64,65,66, 68,73,80,81,94,95,99,100
Pegfilgrastim	18
Pemetrexed	12
Pentostatin	15
Physical activity	2
Phytonutrients	2-4, 6,30
Pineapple	18-20,25,27,82,104,118,124
Potassium	12-13,18
Potatoes	10,12,21,28,29,40,44, 72,75,76,87,98,101,105
Pralatrexate	14
Prednisone	18
Preventive nutrition	9,11
Procarbazine	12,15
Protein	3,6,8,9,12,14-16, 18-20,22,24,27,28,30
Protein powder	6,8,9,19,24,30,116,124-131, 133-138,141-143
Purinethol	16
Radiation	8,9,11,19,22,27
Raloxifene	14
Rapamycin	16
Raspberries	2,21,27,30,137
Regenerative nutrition	6
Revlimid	16
Rituxan	16
Rituximab	16
Roferon	16
Sandostatin	16
Selenium	6,22,25
Sirolimus	16
Smoking	2,22
Sorafenib	15
Spinach	3,4,21,25,28,29,45, 48,93,97,102,103
Sprycel	16
St. John's Wort	21
Strawberries	21,25,111,122,130,140,141,143
Streptozocin	17
Sunitinib	16
Surgery	8,20-22
Sutent	16
Swallowing difficulties	22
Tamoxifen	16
Tarceva	16
Targretin	16
Tasigna	16
Taxol	12,16
Taxotere	16
Temodar	16
Temozolomide	16

Temsirolimus 17
Teniposide 17
TESPA 16
Testosterone 13-14
Thalidomide 17
Thalomid 17
TheraCys 17
Thioguanine 17
6-Thioguanine 17
Thiotepa 16
Tomatoes 4,7,21,22,25,29,35,38,
           41,43,48,49,51,53,61,64,75,
           81,83,94,95,104,106,107
Toposar 17
Topotecan 14
Toremifene 14
Torisel 17
Tositumomab 13
Trastuzumab 14
Treanda 17
Trexall 17
Tribulus terrestris 13,14
Trisenox 17
Turmeric 9,13,15,21,27,30
Tykerb 17
Valerian 21
VCR 17
Vectibix 17
Velban 17
Velcade, bortezomib, BZM 17
VePesid 17
Vesanoid 17
Viadur 17
Vinblastine 17
Vincristine 15,17
Vinorelbine tartrate 15

Vitamin A 6,8,12,17,24,35,41,43,49,52,
           66,67,71,74,75,78,91,99,102,
           106-108,111,116,120,124,125,
           127,129,133,134,135,139,142
Vitamin B2 25,56,60,61,62,63,
           77,79,85,88,90,106
Vitamin B6 25,44,46,50,51,54,55,57,59,
           60,66,68,69,71,72,80,86,87,
           88,89,90,91,95,98,101,105,
           108,116,142
Vitamin C 4,8,25,35-38,41,42,45,46,48-51,
           53,55,56,59,61,62,64,65,68,69,
           70,72,73,74,77,79-85,94-105,
           107,111,115,117-121,125-129,
           132-136,138,140-143
Vitamin E 3,22,25
Vitamin K 18
Vomiting 23
VP-16 17
Vumon 17
Walnuts 3,7,14,21,22,26,28,89,112
Xeloda 17
Zanosar 17
Zinecard 18
Zevalin 17
Zinc 2,6,13,25,30,36,42,44-46,48,
           52-57,59-71,77,79-82,85,89,
           90,94,97,103,106,108,111,116,
           125-127,130,131,133-136,138,
           141-143
Zoledronic acid 17
Zoladex 17
Zometa 17

BIBLIOGRAPHY and FURTHER READING

Books and Publications

American Cancer Society Textbook of Clinical Oncology, 4th Edition. Editors Arthur I. Holleb, Diane J. Fink, Gerald Patrick Murphy Nutrition for the Chemotherapy Patient, Janet Ramstack, DrPH and Ernest H. Rosenbaum, MD. Bull Publishing, 1990

Nutritional Oncology, 2nd Edition. Editors George L. Blackburn, Bay Lian W. Go, John Milner and David Heber. Academic Press, 2006

The Omega Plan, Artemis Simopoulos, MD and Jo Robinson. Harper Collins, 1998

The Wellness Community Guide to Fighting for Recovery from Cancer, Harold H. Benjamin, PhD. Tarcher Putnam, 1995 (The first edition of this book is Appendix 1

Radiation Therapy and You: Support for People with Cancer. National Cancer Institute publication #P123, 2010 also online at www.nci.gov

Chemotherapy and You: Support for People with Cancer. National Cancer Institute publication #P117, 2008 also online at www.nci.gov

Eating Hints: Before, During and After Cancer Treatment. National Cancer Institute publication #P118, 2011 also online at www.nci.gov

The EVERYTHING Cancer Fighting Cookbook. by Carolyn Katzin, MS, CNS, MNT Adams Media, 2010

Nutrition and physical activity during and after cancer treatment: an American Cancer Society guide for informed choices. CA Cancer J Clin. 2003 Sep-Oct; 53(5):268-91. Brown JK, Byers T, Doyle C, Coumeya KS, Demark-Wahnefried W, Kushi LH, McTieman A, Rock CL, Aziz N, Bloch AS, Eldridge B, Hamilton K, Katzin C, Koonce A, Main J, Mobley C, Morra ME, Pierce MS, Sawyer KA; American Cancer Society

Organizations and Resource Websites

American Cancer Society www.cancer.org
American College of Nutrition www.americancollegeofnutrition.org
American Dietetic Association www.eatright.org
American Institute for Cancer Research www.aicr.org
American Society for Nutrition www.nutrition.org
Certification Board of Nutrition Specialists www.cbns.org
Memorial Sloan-Kettering Cancer Center www.mskcc.org on herbs & botanicals
National Cancer Institute www.cancer.gov

Cancer Nutrition Center www.cancernutrition.com